D0404191

STATIN DRUGS SIDE EFFECTS
and the Misguided War on Cholesterol

By
Duane Graveline, M.D.

Copyright © 2004 - 2008 by Duane Graveline, M.D.

Published by: Duane Graveline, M.D.

First published - November, 2004

4th Edition – Fifth Printing - May, 2008

Printed in the United States of America.

ACKNOWLEDGEMENT

To all my friends and colleagues in the medical, health, nutrition and research professions whose knowledge and guidance have paved the way to my writing this book, my gratitude is endless. Your encouragement and advice were essential ingredients to its becoming.

But the most profound encouragement for my bringing these unknown and often obscure cognitive, neuromuscular and behavioral side effects of the statin drugs to public attention comes from the letters I have received from thousands of patients, their families and concerned friends, here in our country and around the world. Their almost desperate need to understand what has happened or was happening to them and why was a powerful incentive - especially in the denial or ignorance of these many different side effects by their doctors and other health caregivers. So many of these victims have related how learning about my experience with transient global amnesia v spacedoc.net has helped relieve the stress and anxiety about their own concerns. I hope this book fulfills their expectations for more complete information about the true legacy of statin drugs as currently used and guidance towards alternative therapies, when indicated.

Duane Graveline, M.D.

CONTENTS

CHAPTER 1
How the Statin Drugs Work?

The development of statin drugs was an almost inevitable phenomenon. After decades of concentrating on cholesterol as the supposed culprit in arteriosclerosis and atherosclerosis, the pharmaceutical community wasn't about to waste its time and resources looking for anything, except the simplest way to "cut it off at the pass."

The biogenesis of cholesterol starts from a simple chemical reaction: Under the influence of ultraviolet radiation, photosynthetic plants combine water with carbon dioxide, the well-known gas we exhale in every breath, to form glucose, the fuel of our bodies.

From this humble origin, the first step toward production of cholesterol in the human body involves the process of glycolosis in which glucose is converted into the two-carbon molecule, building blocks of life known as Acetyl-CoA. These simple fragments then combine to start the cholesterol biosynthetic pathway. Next, three molecules of Acetyl-CoA combine stepwise to form the six-carbon hydroxymethyl glutaric acid part of the intermediate complex known as HMG-CoA, which has proven to be the Achilles heel of cholesterol biosynthesis.

This is the weak point in the chain of events the pharmaceutical industry was looking for and the one that enabled them to develop their statin drugs, for when two molecules of HMG-CoA next combined to form the ubiquitous mevalonic acid, the enzyme, HMG-CoA reductase was required. This enzyme was quite easily inhibited and suddenly a multibillion-dollar industry was born with the development of the HMG-CoA reductase inhibitors known as the statin drugs. Whether Lipitor®, Mevacor®, Zocor®, Pravachol®, Crestor®, Vytorin®, Lescol®, or the ill-fated Baycol®, all use the same mechanism and are merely variations of the same theme as marketed by different pharmaceutical companies to obtain market share.

Research biochemists soon identified the HMG-CoA reductase step as a natural control point for cholesterol synthesis since the reaction was not reversible and it was the slowest step of the entire cholesterol pathway. It seemed a natural point for cholesterol control - the pharmaceutical companies now had their "corral." One can almost feel the pulse of industry leaders quicken in anticipation of the potential market size.

Cholesterol, discovered as a major constituent of gallstones, was identified in 1775 as the first known steroid. As a steroid, it is a member of the vast array of natural products known as the terpenoids. Man has used these substances since antiquity as ingredients of flavors, preservatives, perfumes, medicines, narcotics, soaps and pigments. By 1894 the name terpene was derived from research into the manufacture of camphor from turpentine. The relationship of steroids to the terpenoids was not discovered until the late 1950's. Since then the modern study of cholesterol has included some of the most creative and productive scientists of the twentieth century. The biosynthesis of cholesterol was worked out by the biochemists Konrad Bloch, Rudolph Schoenheimer, Fyodor Lynen and many others. Bloch, who received the Nobel Prize in 1964, was Kilmer McCully's professor and mentor at Harvard, helping to guide the promising young biochemist and beginning pathologist along his future path of elucidating homocysteine's role in the etiology of arteriosclerosis. The research on the biosynthesis of cholesterol continues undiminished today. Scientists marvel at the astonishing efficiency and sheer elegance of the steroid biosynthetic pathway. Its complexity is such as to nearly defy human credulity.

The mevalonic acid-HMG-CoA reductase step is but the first step on the long climb to cholesterol synthesis. Many intermediate steps are required before the ultimate goal of cholesterol synthesis is achieved. In at least two of these steps, five carbon units of the enormous steroid class of drugs, destined to be used for other biosynthetic pathways in the human body, are involved. Statin drugs, while curtailing cholesterol biosynthesis, must inevitably inhibit the production of these vital intermediary products, primary among which are ubiquinone (Co-enzyme Q10)[1] and dolichols. One might say these unavoidable, collateral consequences might yet prove to be the Achilles heel of the statin drugs, in that the side effects resulting from impaired production of these substances are intolerable, harmful and even lethal to many people.

The pharmaceutical industry has long been attempting to develop a means by which interference with cholesterol production might be achieved farther along the biosynthetic pathway, beyond the point where these vital intermediary products originate but up to now, have failed. There is reason to believe that such biochemical maneuvering, even if successful for restoring such vital intermediary substances as ubiquinone and dolichols, may be completely inadequate to address the full spectrum of physiological consequences from statin drug use. Certainly any hormonal consequences from inadequate cholesterol availability, such as testosterone and progesterone deficiency, would remain an issue. And, as Pfreiger has so brilliantly demonstrated, impairment of synapse formation and function in our brain cells from deficient cholesterol manufacture by our glial cells would continue unabated. Additionally, even if the dedicated researchers of the pharmaceutical industry discover a way around these two, very substantial side effects, even greater hurdles exist from our recent evidence that statins work not by cholesterol manipulation but by some basic anti-inflammatory role[2,3,4,5,6].

Key to this is a substance known as nuclear factor kappa B. All statins inhibit this vital step in our immune system's ability to defend us from alien forces. Whether by being the recipient of a donor kidney or under attack by bacteria or viruses, our immune system has evolved a defensive strategy in which inflammation, triggered by nuclear factor kappa B (NF-kB), plays a vital role. Such stimulants to inflammation include the foreign sclerotic and thrombotic changes in our arteries from arterial wall damage. Statin drugs are now known to suppress this nuclear factor kappa B response and thereby open a veritable Pandora's box of unpredictable consequences. [7]

So we have then several different mechanisms of action of the statin class of drugs. The first is cholesterol reduction, a task our statins accomplish with great effectiveness in most people. Unfortunately we now are learning that this cholesterol manipulation is irrelevant to atherosclerosis and increased cardiovascular risk. The second action of statins is to inhibit NF-kB and this appears to be the secret to its remarkable effectiveness in cardiovascular risk reduction. The third action of statin is a consequence of this NK-kB inhibition, that of altering the effectiveness of our immuno-defense system[8,9,10,11]. The fourth is that of ubiquinone inhibition with its extraordinary consequences relevant to energy production[12,13,14,15] and cell wall integrity[16] and the fifth is dolichol inhibition with its own broad range of potential behavioral manifestations.

This sobering information as to the full scope of statin drug's potential side effects is completely new to the practicing physicians, most of whom are still trying to cope with the somewhat better understood reality of muscle pain and hepatic inflammation.

And mention must be given to the over the counter statin, bearing the name, Red Yeast Rice. This substance has been around for over 3,000 years and is Mother Nature's purely natural statin, derived by the fermentation of rice. Its active ingredient is lovastatin. Each 600 mg capsule of Red Yeast Rice contains roughly 2 mg of lovastatin, the same active ingredient that is in Merck's Mevacor. Although Merck, the developer of Mevacor, was predictably concerned about the potential of this entirely natural substance to compete with their product, it is on the shelves of most health food stores as a dependable product. As to its potency, there have been many cases of myopathy associated with its use and at least one case of rhabdomyolysis.

One of the more tragic case reports from our unfortunate statin past comes from Steve Sparks,[17] the well-known statin activist. He reports that his father prided himself on doing whatever he could to stay healthy. At the time of being prescribed Baycol®, this octogenarian was totally self-supportive, very active in church activities and walked up to 4 miles a day.

He was prescribed Baycol® at 0.8 mg on 6 December 2000 for mildly elevated cholesterol and had no other significant medical problems. Within 24 days, he was hospitalized with complete renal failure and a CPK of 150,000. He died 24 January 2001. On 10 August 2001, Steve Sparks filed a class action suit against Bayer and began his current role as statin drug activist, determined that what had happened to his father should never again happen to any patient.

Despite the belated withdrawal of Baycol, rhabdomyolysis deaths still occur because all currently used statin drugs share the ubiquinone depleting side effect of Baycol, although to a lesser degree. Also relevant are the growing number of reports in the literature of biopsy proven myositis in many patient having muscle soreness unheralded by muscle enzyme elevations telling us that despite reassurances of the drug industry and industry sponsored research, prescribing physicians would be wise to be cautious. The continuing problem of rhabdomyolysis due to statin drugs other than Baycol® is best exemplified by the following case report on file both with FDA's Medwatch and in Dr. Beatrice Golomb's statin study at the University of California San Diego, College of Medicine.[18]

The CEO of a large company began to take Lipitor® in 1998 at the time of an emergency angioplasty. His recovery and subsequent course was unremarkable until the past year when two things happened to make this 54-year old man both the luckiest and unluckiest man to come to our attention. Generalized muscle pain ushered in his bad luck, and the diagnosis was severe rhabdomyolysis manifested by extensive muscle cell breakdown, rising muscle enzyme levels and profound secondary blockage of the kidney tubules by damaged muscle cell debris. Associated with this condition was the loss of respiratory control during

11

sleep and the loss of his ability to express or understand ideas. A physical work-up revealed the usual findings associated with severe rhabdomyolysis muscle cell breakdown but it also included the somewhat surprising presence of a profound loss of short-term memory. "Odd" memory glitches had occurred during the preceding year but he had passed them off as due to lack of concentration. His good luck has been the resourcefulness and support of his wife and family.

He barely survived the rhabdomyolysis and still suffers constant pain and weakness, but his major problem is persistent and probably permanent cognitive impairment. According to his wife his doctors concur that the damage was somehow caused by Lipitor®, a likelihood supported by the failure of extensive testing to show the presence of tumors, stroke or even Alzheimer's. His Lipitor® was stopped on 19 January 2002.

The most alarming episode of this man's transient global amnesia occurred in April of 2002, three months after Lipitor® was discontinued. He experienced a "flashback" reaction comparable to the one that sometimes occurs months after a drug overdose. On 4 April 2002, as his wife left for work, he volunteered to go to the local store for groceries and, after noting the progressive "greening" of their swimming pool, added he would pick up some chlorine as well. He did the grocery shopping with the aid of his new palm pilot and several cell phone calls to his wife about dinner items for the coming weekend. He then went to The

Home Depot® to pick up the chlorine and a few other small hardware items. When he parked the car in The Home Depot parking lot he decided to transfer his frozen foods to the trunk before going inside. When he opened the trunk the chlorine and the other items he was planning to buy were sitting there in a The Home Depot shopping bag. The experience greatly upset him, since he had absolutely no recall of going into Home Depot and buying the items. To add to his befuddlement, when his wife arrived home that evening and checked the receipts, they discovered that the Home Depot chlorine purchase had been made the previous day. No one had been home the previous day when he took out his classic convertible, drove to his errand, and then returned home with absolutely no recollection. He was devastated.

When the reality of his memory impairment became clear, other unusual 'memory' lapses were recalled. One of these odd events had occurred almost a year before stopping Lipitor® when, while on an errand, he suddenly realized that he was inexplicably heading north on the freeway far away from, and in the wrong direction for, anything he had intended to do. This episode bothered him but he passed it off as preoccupation.

Another odd event had occurred on 27 December 2001 while they were at their lakeshore camp a few weeks before his life threatening rhabdomyolysis occurred. He had left the house at approximately 4:30 am to do some shore fishing, returning at approximately 8:30 am. When asked if he went fishing he could not recall and was clearly flustered, embarrassed and thoroughly upset over his inability to remember. His wife adds that he must have gone fishing since there is nothing else to do for 40 miles in either direction.

His wife then recalled on 2 January 2002, while he was still on Lipitor®, he had called her on his cell phone when she was on her way to work. He wanted to know why he was in The Home Depot parking lot. He was not sure why he was there and was flustered, embarrassed and upset not to know. She also recalled that in November and December of 2001 he started some woodworking projects to be used for gifts. After the projects were completed, he would still go into the garage and find wood components already cut, proof that he had restarted the project several times, evidentially forgetting that he had already completed them.

She recorded additional post-Lipitor® observations and realized an episode of aberrant behavior occurred on 22 Mar 2002 that fit the TGA profile. Her upset husband had called her at work, from their home, and commented that it had been a bad day. He started out in the morning to go to the office and then to the bank and had placed the banking items on the seat of his car. When he arrived back at home he realized that they were still on the seat so he took the car out again to go to the bank. He set out on the freeway and forgot where he was going. He recalled that when he suddenly looked down and discovered that he was nearly out of gas, he pulled off the freeway and filled the tank.

However, at that point he had no idea why he had even been on the freeway or where he was going. It frightened him so much that he went straight home and determined not to leave the house again that day. When told about this, his daughter commented she had seen him on the road and waved at him. He had looked right at her face while she was waving but had not responded. He had no memory of seeing her or her very distinctive car and, since his car was equally distinctive, the chance of either of them making a mistake is very small.

Since 4 April 2002, no further transient global amnesia-like episodes have been noted. This formerly successful CEO is now "cognitively impaired" and unable to work, testing below the 1st percentile for short-term memory and cognition. He has been off Lipitor® for almost six months with little or no improvement in his short-term memory and his case is one of the rare, reported instances of persistent and possibly permanent cognitive disturbance associated with statin drug use.

Of special interest is the fact that three uneventful years passed before this CEO's Lipitor®-associated problems surfaced in the form of his first "memory lapse," and another year was to pass before the dreaded complication of rhabdomyolysis began. This is a sobering observation for those who would seek comfort from the fact that they have been taking a statin drug for a year with no problem. The relationship of this executive's apparently permanent short-term memory loss to the rhabdomyolysis remains to be determined. One would surmise that permanent damage to the memory apparatus must have occurred, particularly to the hippocampal area, yet neurologic studies have failed to demonstrate the lesion - an enigma, it would seem.

The statin drugs are in widespread use today and the trend to promote their use even more broadly seems inevitable at present, particularly when one considers the proliferating TV commercial exposure. One doctor, extremely skeptical that cognitive side effects could be associated with statin drug use, claimed that the only problem with statins lies in the fact that they are not getting to everyone who needs them.

Currently most practicing physicians feel that the statins are the best drugs available for high-risk stroke and heart attack patients and are clearly to be recommended when more conservative measures such as diet and exercise are inadequate. There is no doubt that statin drugs substantially reduce cholesterol levels in most people, but there is growing concern among researchers reporting on major clinical trials that cholesterol reduction is not leading to significant reductions in cardiovascular disease mortality.[19,20,21]

Even when statin therapy does seem to increase survival in CHD patients as reported by Collins, et al, for a large group of diabetics and non-diabetics treated with simvastatin for occlusive arterial disease[22], one must be wary of the confusing and often misleading use of statistics presented in many randomized controlled trials. For a masterful discussion of the use of statistics to confuse the reader and inflate the true benefit of statin therapy, one need only read Dr. Uffe Ravnskov's book, The Cholesterol Myths[23]. Additionally in his book, Ravnskov reported of the recent PROSPER trial published in Lancet, that statin therapy increased the incidence of cancer deaths, completely offsetting the slight decrease in deaths from cardiovascular disease and further complicating interpretation of reported benefits from statin therapy. Most researchers feel this increased number of cancer deaths is based on compromise of our immunodefence system due to NF-kB inhibition.

This observation of increased cancer deaths associated with statin drug use and forecast of more to come was stressed by Paul Rosch MD in his Weston-Price Foundation review presentation of May 2003[24]. Support for his concern is evident in the Japan Lipid Intervention Trial observation[25] of excess deaths from malignancy in their so called statin "hyper-responders", that sub-group of patients whose total serum cholesterols plummeted to less than 160 mg % during the study period. Of the 12 cancer deaths reported, four were from gastric cancer and 2 were from lung cancer, This heightened cancer risk almost certainly is based on loss of immuno-resistance secondary to inhibition of NK- kB, mentioned earlier in this chapter although other factors may play a role.

Because of this growing specter of doubt about the effectiveness of cholesterol reduction on cardiovascular disease and the risks inherent in statin drug use, there is very real concern about the escalating use of these drugs for primary prevention. Despite a diligent search of the literature, one can find remarkably little support for broader use of the statins for cholesterol reduction. Moderate hypercholesterolemics - with or without diabetes, obesity, smoking history, hypertension or a family history of the disease - who are now being placed on statin drugs because "everyone knows they are effective and safe", may be better treated by alternative means or by dramatically lowered statin doses.

The physiological implications of these drugs are profound when based on just what is actually known at this time, but when one adds the reality of our present shallow grasp of physiology at the intracellular and molecular level, there is justification for the question, "Do we really know what we are doing?"

So the mechanism of action of the statin class of drugs is far from simple inhibition of cholesterol bio-synthesis. In reality the statin drugs have now been proven to have five distinct faces and even more are likely to be found as our research continues. The first face of statins is that of cholesterol reduction. This is a task they do with great efficiency. Lipitor, Zocor and its offspring, Vytorin take pride in causing up to 40% reduction of total serum cholesterol in many people. The newcomer to the statin scene, Crestor, goes much further with respect to inhibition of cholesterol biosynthesis, claiming as much as 52 % reduction in many people. But now the results of our long-term studies are revealing some remarkable truths. Cholesterol, our nemesis for the past four decades in our fight against cardiovascular disease, has now achieved a position in causality remarkably close to irrelevant. Inflammation is the cause of heightened cardiovascular risk, our researchers are now telling us! Cholesterol is innocent in its physiologically natural form. Cholesterol is drawn passively into the atherosclerotic plaque by "misguided" LDL. Even our "misguided" LDL may not be LDL at all but a structurally similar substance, known as lipoprotein (a), having a radically different physiological effect. Natural cholesterol is not the cause of our infamous atherosclerotic plaques.

We now have proven that atherosclerosis is the result of inflammatory factors such as homocysteine, secondary to genetic or acquired deficiencies of vitamin B6, B12 and folic acid. Homocysteine has been shown to be a major player in atherosclerotic change, with coagulation defects, platelet factors, omega-6 and selected anti-oxidant deficiencies responsible for most of the rest. Cholesterol no longer is deserving of even a place in the lineup of usual suspects.

It was only in 2003 that Pfrieger[26] found that the glial cells of the brain provide for brain cholesterol manufacture and of course are just as effectively inhibited by statins, finally giving an explanation for our bizarre cognitive side effects being reported, our first face of statins' pleotrophic effects. Now we had a mechanism for our amnesia, confusion, disorientation, forgetfulness and aggravation of pre-existing senility – the lack of sufficient bioavailability of cholesterol for proper neuronal function. And we must heed particularly the findings of Muldoon[27] that one can document cognitive deterioration in 100% of statin users with the right type of testing.

So now we know the second face of statin drugs, the effective face, the face that no doubt has prevented many cases of heart attacks and strokes. No one seriously argues the positive effects of this happy face but it is anti-inflammatory, not cholesterol lowering. It is a face only recently recognized as the results of long-term studies have been analyzed. Whether your cholesterol goes up, down or remains unchanged, statin drugs work by a means independent of cholesterol. This factor is nuclear factor-kappa B, a transcriptase common to our entire immuno-defense system.

The entire pharmaceutical industry has been shocked by this revelation but quick to acknowledge and adapt to the change for now statins are being promoted for organ transplant recipients and as adjunctive therapy in the treatment of auto-immune diseases. Why? Because they work! These results are sobering, indeed, for statin drugs can work in this capacity only at the risk of causing mischief elsewhere.

The third face of statin drug effect is this same nuclear factor-kappa B and its effect on the remainder of our immune system? What about cancer and infectious disease? We have had 3.5

billion years to work out our defense systems against widely diverse challenges and NF-kB is key to all of them. Whether by being the recipient of a donor kidney or under attack by bacteria or viruses, or having a mutation induced by radiation in our environment, our immune system has evolved a defensive strategy in which suppression of inflammation, triggered by nuclear factor kappa B, plays a vital role. The ability of statin drugs to suppress this nuclear factor kappa B response is potentially to confound the inner workings of our entire immuno-defense system.

Ubiquinone deficiency is the fourth face of statins and the one responsible for our most severe side effects. Statin drugs, while curtailing cholesterol, must inevitably inhibit the production of other vital intermediary products that originate further down the metabolic pathway beyond the statin blockade. The pharmaceutical industry has long been attempting to develop a means by which interference with cholesterol production might be achieved beyond the point where these vital intermediary products originate but up to now have failed. The inevitability of significant, serious and even lethal side effects has been knowingly accepted. Ubiquinone levels plummet when statins are initiated.

Such side effects, as congestive heart failure and chronic fatigue, reflect ubiquinone's important role in energy production. Hepatitis, myopathy, rhabdomyolysis and peripheral neuropathy reflect ubiquinone's role in cell wall integrity and stability.

Ubiquinone's role in the prevention of somatic mitochondrial mutations also is of critical importance and introduces a vast area of concern.

The fifth face of statin drug effect has to do with dolichol availability. Like the ubiquinones, this class of compounds is inevitably collaterally damaged with statin drug use, for it branches off the same biosynthetic tree. Dolichols are vital to our intricate process of neuropeptide formation. Neuropeptides are biochemicals that regulate almost all life processes on a cellular level, thereby linking all body systems. Although produced primarily in the brain, every cell in the body produces and exchanges neuropeptides, Called messenger molecules, they send chemical messages in the form of linked peptides from the brain to receptor sites on cell membranes throughout the body. Every thought, sensation and emotion we have ever felt has been dependent upon the makeup of these peptide linkages and, surprisingly, they do not simply convey. These peptide clusters are the thought, sensation or emotion in a process we are only just beginning to understand.

We now strongly suspect disruption of this system by statins is behind our reports of depression, irritability, hostility, aggressiveness, road rage type behavior, accident and addiction proneness and our reports of suicides soon after statin drugs are started.

When confronted by the reality that one's statin is causing intolerable, even dangerous, side effects the question of alternatives or stopping one's statin inevitably arises. A frequent course of action is to try another statin but only rarely does this resolve the problem for all statins are HMG Co-A reductase inhibitors and as such work only in one way – to inhibit the reductase step on the mevalonate pathway of cholesterol biosynthesis. So if you are experiencing muscle pain, short term memory loss, unusual tiredness or depression with your new statin and change to another statin seems futile, what then?

For one who is experiencing the sudden onset of myopathy with rapid progression the answer is obvious - the offending statin is stopped immediately but for most symptoms time is not critical and the patient has a choice. Logically, patients might ask, "How should I stop my statin, cold turkey, gradual or what?" The problem I see is that increasingly I am receiving case reports saying, "I have heard of the side effects of statins in the media (or seen it in a Forum while Internet browsing), my symptoms are the same. I have stopped my statin and wonder what I should do about my high cholesterol?"

To understand my response, you must understand statins' vital role in reduction of cardiovascular disease risk. Cholesterol has nothing to do with this. Statins' impressive benefits are due solely to their anti-inflammatory action, their powerful ability to inhibit nuclear factor kappa B. This substance is vital to our immune system's function of triggering an inflammatory response to disease. As I mentioned earlier in this book, statins work their magic of lowering cardiovascular disease risk not by cholesterol reduction but by their inherent anti-inflammatory action. Monocyte adhesion, macrophage recruitment, smooth muscle migration and platelet activation are all parts of our body's defensive inflammatory response, even if such inflammation occurs within the walls of our blood vessels as part of the process of atherosclerosis. Platelet activation is essential to this response to help seal off the disease regardless of its cause. Statins' inhibition of NF-kB reduces the likelihood of thrombosis with our blood vessels during this inflammatory assault, hence its undeniable record in reducing the degree of atherosclerosis and CV risk. You might recall that aspirin has a similar but far less aggressive effect on platelet function.

Now let us assume you have been on a statin for a few months or years during which time it has provided inhibition of inflammatory activity within your blood vessels. That's good. But then you experience memory loss or severe myopathy and must come off statins. When this is done, there is a return of normal platelet activation (stickiness) in most people but some recent studies have shown there will be an overshoot of platelet stickiness, peaking in the second week after stopping the statin. The result is a small but significant tendency for strokes and infarctions to occur during that time. The obvious solution is a gradual tapering off of statins, not abrupt cessation.

My strong recommendation, then, is that a statin user who has made the decision to stop his or her statin must do so gradually over at least a two-week period. Pill cutters are invaluable for this process. For example, someone on Lipitor 40mg will cut to 20 for a few days, then 10 for a few days, then 5 and 2.5mg. In this manner any peaking of platelet stickiness will be avoided. I might add that buffered aspirin 81mg during this tapering off phase will be helpful and will also be an important part of your alternative treatment plan of omega-3, CoQ10 and vitamins B6, 12 and folic acid as discussed in my statin alternatives chapter.

How strange it is that a class of drugs developed solely for the purpose of interfering with the biosynthesis of cholesterol has now been shown to reduce cardiovascular risk by a novel and unsuspected anti-inflammatory role completely unrelated to cholesterol manipulation. We now have a nation of patients and doctors convinced that cholesterol is public health enemy number one, for none of this recent truth has yet significantly penetrated the hallowed halls of health care delivery. A patient's first question when told his mental aberration is most likely a side effect of a statin will say, "But what can I do about my cholesterol?"

We have a pharmaceutical industry still committed to pushing the charade of cholesterol etiology. Imagine the billions of profit dollars resulting to them from perpetuating the myth of cholesterol? Now, when confronted by the reality of inflammation, they deftly turn their sights towards organ transplant and auto-immune disease.

Perhaps stockholder loyalty explains why Pfizer management knew over a decade ago, during the first human use trial of Lipitor, of the cognitive impact to come when Lipitor was released to the public. Of their 2503 patients tested with Lipitor, seven experienced transient global amnesia attacks and four others experienced other forms of severe memory disturbances, for a total of 11 cases out of 2,503 test patients. This is a ratio of five cases of severe cognitive loss to result from every 1000 patients that took the drug. Not one word of warning of this was ever transmitted to the thousands of physicians who soon would be dispensing the drug. This greatly helps to explain why, when I asked about FAA's allowance of statin drug use in commercial airline pilots, one[28] of FAA's leading flight surgeons told me, "I did not know statins could do this."

Today with 30 million patients on Lipitor and using Pfizer's own data, we can expect an astounding 150,000 cases of severe cognitive loss this year alone.

CHAPTER 2
Statins and Brain Cholesterol

Pfreiger's announcement on 9 November 2001 about the discovery of the identity of the elusive synaptogenic factor responsible for the development of synapses, the highly specialized contact sites between adjacent neurons in the brain[1], deserves to be cited again in the context of cholesterol's vast importance to our bodies. Not surprisingly to specialists in the field, the synaptogenic factor was shown to be the notorious substance cholesterol!

The so-called glial cells, the non-nervous or supporting tissue of the brain and spinal cord long suspected of providing certain housekeeping functions, were shown to produce their own supply of cholesterol for the specific purpose of providing nerve cells with this vital synaptic component. As many of you may know, the neuronal synapse of the nervous system is the basis of neurotransmission connecting the brain with the rest of the body. The brain cannot tap the cholesterol supply in the blood because the lipoproteins that carry cholesterol - both LDL and HDL - in the blood are too large to pass the blood-brain barrier[2]. The brain must depend upon its own cholesterol synthesis, which the glial cells provide.

This should be sobering news for those in the pharmaceutical industry developing drugs which interfere with cholesterol synthesis, and that is exactly the mechanism of action of all our statins. One wonders how anyone knowing the mechanism of brain cholesterol synthesis can seriously challenge the reality of cognitive side effects from statin drug use. The only surprise is that there are not more reported cases of memory impairment, amnesia, confusion and disorientation.

After nearly five years of letters and e-mails from people regarding statin drug use, I have learned that very few know of the full range of side effects. Even many prescribing physicians are ignorant of the broad reach of the statin class of drugs.

I suppose my first rude awakening of the prevalence of this lack of knowledge among physicians about the drugs they prescribe was during my own personal experience four years ago with transient global amnesia bouts after taking Lipitor. On both occasions, dozens of physicians with whom I came in contact said, "Lipitor doesn't do that."

Dozens of pharmacists during that same time period said the same thing, "Statins don't do that." Now that our statin study has reported nearly one thousand cases of statin associated transient global amnesia, physicians are reluctantly accepting the reality of amnesia, confusion, disorientation, extreme forgetfulness and aggravation of pre-existing senility but many still do not know it exists.

My following personal account has now been replayed hundreds of times in emergency rooms throughout the world as statin users are seen for their amnesias. Mine was one of the first statin associated transient global amnesia (TGA) cases reported to the UCSD statin study six years ago.

"My personal introduction to the incredible world of TGA occurred six weeks after Lipitor® was started during my annual astronaut physical at Johnson Space Center. My cholesterol had been trending upward for several years and all was well until six weeks later when my wife found me aimlessly walking about the yard after I returned from my usual walk in the woods. I did not recognize her, reluctantly accepted cookies and milk and refused to go into my now unfamiliar home. I "awoke" six hours later in the office of the examining neurologist with the diagnosis of transient global amnesia, cause unknown. My MRI several days later was normal. Since Lipitor® was the only new medicine I was on, the doctor in me made me suspect a possible side effect of this drug and, despite the protestations of the examining doctors that statin drugs did not do this, I stopped my Lipitor®.

The year passed uneventfully and soon it was time for my next astronaut physical. NASA doctors joined the chorus I had come to expect from physicians and pharmacists during the preceding year, that statin drugs did not do this and at their bidding I reluctantly restarted Lipitor® at one-half the previous dose. Six weeks later I again descended into the black pit of amnesia, this time for twelve hours and with a retrograde loss of memory back to my high school days. During that terrible interval, when my entire adult life had been eradicated, I had no awareness of my marriage and children, my medical school days, my ten adventure-filled years as a USAF flight surgeon or my selection as NASA scientist astronaut. All had vanished from my mind as completely as if they had never happened. Fortunately, and typically for this obscure condition, my memory returned spontaneously and again I drove home listening to my wife's amazing tale of how my day (and hers) had gone."

The medical literature is now replete with reports of statin associated amnesias and other evidence of mental dysfunction and still many of our prescribing physicians remain unaware of statins' special cognitive impairment tendency.

Their patient's rapid descent into dementia after a statin is started is much too often written off by their doctor as senile brain changes or beginning Alzheimers when the real culprit is their statin drug.

Readers will be interested to know of Muldoon's reports in the medical literature documenting cognitive impairment in 100% of statin users if sufficiently sensitive testing is done[3].

Transient global amnesia is the sudden inability to formulate new memory, known as anterograde amnesia, combined with varying degrees of retrograde memory loss, sometimes for decades into the past[4]. Until recently, the most common trigger events for these abrupt and completely unheralded amnesia cases have been sudden vigorous exercise, sex, emotional crises, cold water immersion, trauma - at times quite subtle, and cerebral angiography. In the past four years a new trigger agent has been added – the use of the stronger statin drugs such as Lipitor®, Zocor® (and its derivative, Vytorin®) and Mevacor®.

Transient global amnesia is but the tip of the iceberg of the many other forms of statin associated memory lapses that are reported from distraught patients[5]. Far more common are symptoms of disorientation, confusion, unusual forgetfulness or increasing senility symptoms. These lesser forms of memory impairment can be easily missed in many individuals because, to a certain degree, that is the nature of us all.

Explanation for a statin drug's effect on our cognition first came on 9 November 2001, when Dr. Pfreiger of the Max Planck Society for the Advancement of Science announced to the world that without abundant supplies of cholesterol, normal synaptic function cannot take place. To refresh your memory, synapses are the connection between our neurons. Our neurons are what we are! It is not surprising that Muldoon reported 100% cognitive loss in statin users if sufficiently sensitive testing is done. We are not precise creatures and most of us know it. Few will deny the tendency of our minds for occasional very sketchy recall. Constant vigilance is necessary to keep us from "wandering".

Knowing the inevitable effect of statins on cholesterol availability to our brains, I sadly shake my head when I read reports where thousands of people were placed on high doses of statins for a special study and their supervising physicians report no significant side effects. In my world, experiencing daily, a constant stream of statin adverse reports, "no significant effects" from that dose of statins is simply not possible!

Charged by nature with the specific task of synthesizing cholesterol for brain function, the glial cells in our brains are just as sensitive to the effect of statins as any other cell in our body. The pharmaceutical industry must have quivered a bit on that surprising news from Pfrieger in 2001 but you would never have known it from their response. They never paused in their aggressive promotion of statins and after five years, they still have not provided any special labeling on drug information pamphlets or verbal warnings by drug "reps" to the thousands of unsuspecting physicians who are prescribing their statin drugs.

So now we have a thoroughly documented mechanism of action for our hundreds of TGA's and other forms of cognitive dysfunction associated with (and possibly even inevitable with) the use of statins. Knowing of this, how is it possible for any responsible physician to say, "Statins don't do this?"

The following are a few "cognitive" reports from the many hundreds of cases in my files:

"Three weeks ago I had an eight-hour episode of TGA. I had been on Lipitor and lisinopril for about six weeks prior. I have stopped both medications for the time being until I get back to normal. Even after stopping the Lipitor I was disoriented (especially in the morning) and "just wasn't feeling right).

32

"Four months ago I was put on Lipitor to reduce my bad cholesterol to 100. Suddenly I found I could not handle basic math or remember how to spell. It became so bad that I was in a constant fog. I should tell you I spent most of my career in Silicon Valley writing specifications for software and hold a patent on expert system technology. I had an MRI to rule out a brain tumor or stroke. Since the only thing that had changed was the addition of Lipitor I stopped taking it. Five weeks later I am still having problems spelling and frequently forget things."

"I am a woman, now 64 years old. I was put on Mevacor after a heart attack in November 2001. At the time my cholesterol level was about 185. After about two years, I read of the possibility of memory loss associated with this medicine. I had been increasingly worried as I was finding that I was forgetting customers' orders, which was very surprising, as I had always had an excellent memory. I discontinued the Mevacor in February of 2004, and in about two weeks noticed that not only was my mind more clear but severe pain and mobility loss that I had been having in my arms was much improved; a hand tremor that had recently become apparent disappeared completely, and a cataract that had become much worse over those two years was improved about to its previous level. Now a year later, I have regained most of the range of motion in my arms and rarely have the muscle pain. At last check my cholesterol level was 235, higher than when the whole thing started."

CHAPTER 3
Statins and CoQ10

We must next consider the impaired production of our vital ubiquinone coenzyme, a collaterally damaged area of great concern since the biochemical ramifications are both broad and profound. Ubiquinone is arguably our most important essential nutrient[1]. Its role in energy production is to make possible the transfer of electrons from one protein complex to another within the inner membrane of our mitochondria to its ultimate recipient, ATP. The adult human body pool of this substance has been reported to be 2 grams and requires replacement of about 0.5 grams per day[2]. This must be supplied by endogenous synthesis or dietary intake. Synthesis decreases progressively in humans above age 21 and the average ubiquinone content of the western diet is less than 5 mg/day. Thus, ubiquinone supplementation appears to be the only way for older people to obtain their daily need of this important nutrient. Nearly 30 million people will be taking Lipitor this year in the United States alone with an additional 20 million taking other types of statin drugs of comparable effect. Most of these people will be over 50 years of age. Few of them will be on supplemental ubiquinone. Simple logic dictates that the statin drug impact on ubiquinone availability and mitochondrial energy production will be profound!

Because of the extremely high-energy demands of the heart, this organ is usually the first to feel statin-associated CoQ10 depletion as cardiomyopathy and congestive heart failure. The importance of mitochondrial function in meeting the energy needs of the heart has been emphasized recently because of the increasing tendency for congestive heart failure (CHF) in statin drug users[3]. Peter Langsjoen, well-known cardiologist, has published a series of excellent articles on this subject[4] and reviewed the prevalence of statin associated CHF in many controlled studies, reporting on the prompt response of CHF to supplemental ubiquinone or reductions in statin dosage.

Perhaps it should be added here that the heart as an organ is just another striated muscle, presumably subject to the same statin-related pathology as the rhabdomyolysis of muscles in general. But the cardiomyopathy of congestive heart failure seems based primarily in the depletion of energy reserves at the mitochondrial level. However, both myopathy in general and cardiomyopathy relate strongly to statin drug depletion of coenzyme Q10 reserves.

Ubiquinone in a slightly altered form known as ubiquinol is found in all membranes where it has a vital function in maintaining membrane integrity. Liver inflammation, with breakdown of liver cells releasing their enzymes into the blood stream and thereby serving as a marker of statin damage, is likely due, at least in part, to loss of cell wall integrity. Breakdown of cell walls secondary to excessive ubiquinol inhibition by statin drug use is suspected to be involved in both the neuropathy and myopathy case reports now flooding the literature. Myopathy, if sufficiently severe may lead to rhabdomyolysis, a condition wherein muscle cell walls break down and release myoglobin causing secondary blockage of kidney tubules. Baycol was removed from the market primarily on the basis of excessive tendency for muscle cell damage and breakdown. Unfortunately, many deaths resulted before this corrective action was taken. And have rhabdomyolysis deaths now disappeared? The answer is no, for it is inherent in all statins. Patients still die from this statin side effect on muscles but at lower rates, less irritating to FDA's eyes, perhaps but still grossly irritating to mine in view of cholesterol's irrelevancy in cardiovascular disease risk.

Dr. David Gaist[5] in a study of 116 patients reported a 16 times greater risk of polyneuropathy among long term statin drug users. This new and very serious side effect of statins should be of special concern to diabetics, many of whom have been prescribed statins because of their high-risk status. All doctors know that a very common outcome of long standing diabetes is peripheral neuropathy. To prescribe statins with their established record of neuropathy to these patients because of their special predisposition to heart attack and stroke is a serious decision, a delicate balance of judgment that should be undertaken only after painful soul-searching on the part of the doctor. This is the so-called art of medicine - making the right choice of medicines when considering more than one variable.

And thousands have reported muscle aches and pains from myopathy, the most commonly reported side effect of statin drug use. Some of these have negative tests for CPK[6], representing a growing sub-group of statin damaged cases. Such cases presumably represent a "contained" inflammatory response, wherein muscle cell wall integrity is maintained despite the intracellular turmoil. Many statin users report using muscle discomfort as an indicator of statin dosage and will adjust their statin dose up or down depending on presence or absence of muscle pain. One might call this fool-hardy stunt the equivalent of "dancing with the devil" for they are always right on the edge of serious muscle damage in their efforts to maintain "health."

Ubiquinone is also vital to the formation of elastin and collagen formation. Tendon and ligament inflammation and rupture have frequently been reported by statin drug users and it is likely that the mechanism of this predisposition to damage is related to some yet unknown compromise of ubiquonine's role in connective tissue formation. I have received hundreds of reports reflecting unusual susceptibility of ligaments and tendons to damage while on statin drugs.

There is still another thoroughly documented role for ubiquinone, just as important as mitochondrial energy production and cell wall integrity. That is its role within the mitochondria as a powerful anti-oxidant[7], with a free radical quenching ability some 50 times greater than that of vitamin E. Without adequate stores of ubiquinone and lacking the repair mechanisms common to nuclear DNA, irreversible oxidative damage to mitochondria DNA results from buildup of superoxide and hydroxyl radicals[8]. We must remember that our mitochondria are in immediate contact with oxygen, front line warriors, so to speak, in our struggle to obtain life-giving oxygen without sustaining excessive oxidative damage. The inevitable result of excessive free radical accumulation is an increase in the rate of mitochondrial mutations. According to some the cumulative effect of somatic mitochondrial mutations may contribute directly to many chronic myopathies, diabetes and even aging[8].

Ubiquinone inhibition secondary to the new, stronger class of statin drugs is well known to the pharmaceutical industry, which has toyed with the idea of recommending that supplemental Coenzyme Q10 be used by patients on statins. Although the drug company Merck obtained a patent for the combination of CoQ10 with statins in one prescribed dose, no further action was ever taken on this matter.

This oversight by Merck laid the groundwork for Dr. Sidney Wolfe's petition of 20 August 2001[10] and Dr. Julian Whitaker's 23 May 2002 petition[11] with the Food and Drug Administration (FDA).

Dr. Whitaker's petition called on the commissioner of the FDA to change the package insert on all statin drugs and to issue a "black box" warning to consumers of the need to take coenzyme Q10 (CoQ10) whenever they take a statin drug. Of relevance here is the fact that in Canada the Lipitor warning label is strengthened to include warnings not only about CoQ10 depletion but also includes warnings on the closely related L-carnitine deficiencies.

Following are a few additional case reports from my files dealing primarily with excessive inhibition of Coenzyme Q10:

"I am experiencing many of the side effects listed for Lipitor. I have been taking it for quite some time but the worse symptoms are fairly recent. Would this be possible? I have finally been told I have fibromyalgia, which has similar symptoms and problems. Since I read about the fact that Lipitor can be causing muscle problems even when you have a normal CPK I just yesterday stopped taking it to see if it helps. I have muscle and joint pain, cognitive problems, lack of attention, restless leg syndrome, irritable bowel syndrome, problems walking because my hips begin to hurt so badly and extreme fatigue."

"I am 45. When I was in my early 30's my blood levels for cholesterol were measured at over 700. It was so high that they had to dilute my blood to get a

measurement because at the time the readings they were using only went to 400. My trig levels were ~2000 (if memory serves me correctly). I was put on Mevacor at a fairly high dose and my levels only came down to mid-300's. They increased my dosage to the maximum and it came down to the high 200's (280'ish). Soon after taking this level my muscles petered out and my Doc was puzzled. This was very early on in the history of statins and I was one of the first patients that my Doc had that was taking Mevacor at the higher dose. He did some research and had me back off some and add niacin at 3 grams a day. My blood profile looked great for 10 years - 160 total with a 67 HDL; life was good. About 12 months ago things started going south. My levels started to edge back up. I lost my energy and doing simple tasks gave me very sore muscles. I would wake up in the morning all stiff and there were some days were I would not want to even move. The fatigue became so great that I would have a hard time staying awake while driving the 11 miles to work. On the worst days my entire body would be so sore it reminded me of the day after my first day of skiing for the season - but for no reason! My CPK levels have been measure at 313; high but not alarmingly so. However my (new) Doc has told me to taper off my meds until the CPK levels come back down; he does not care about my cholesterol levels at this point. I have been doing research on the web and have found a lot of info indicating that C-Q10 levels could be the real problem. I have taken 200mg for 2 days and I already am starting to feel better. I am still looking for answers but I feel that I am at last on the correct path."

"I just found your web site and am eager to get the new book. I have been taking Lipitor for about a year. Just this week, in preparation for a colonoscopy, the Dr. noticed my liver seemed to be very hard and swollen and scheduled CT Scans of abdomen and pelvic area. I don't have the results yet, but am very concerned that my liver has been damaged. Other side effects including memory loss and muscle pain have been very high, but I had no idea these were side effects of the Lipitor. My doctor prescribed it and never scheduled any follow up blood tests, liver tests, etc. and I did not do the due diligence that I apparently should have."

CHAPTER 4
Statins and Dolichols

Science has amassed so much research knowledge that very little remains simple and straightforward, so one ventures cautiously into the murky complexity of another secondary metabolite potentially compromised by statin drug use - that of the dolichols. The role of dolichols in the manufacture of neuropeptides is an intricate process of cellular activity that has fascinated researchers for years[1]. Neuropeptides are biochemicals that regulate almost all life processes on a cellular level, thereby linking all body systems[2,3,4,5]. Although produced primarily in the brain, every tissue in the body produces and exchanges neuropeptides. Called messenger molecules, they send chemical messages from the brain to receptor sites on cell membranes throughout the body.

Until recently such intercellular information transfer was felt to be the sole province of our classic neurotransmitter chemicals such as serotonin and catecholamines, gate-keepers of our synapses, aided by various hormones carried by our vascular system. Now we have learned that not only do neuropeptides supplement these systems, they provide the vast majority of information transfer. Not only do these protein chains carry information throughout the body, they also mysteriously seem to be the information. They do not simply convey thought, sensation or emotion; these peptide clusters are the thought, sensation or emotion in a process we are only just beginning to understand.

Within each of our cells are miniscule factories of immense complexity. Floating in the cytoplasm is a tubular network of membranes called the endoplasmic reticulum. It is here that peptide units are linked one by one into what amounts to a tiny chain, with the ultimate cellular message of each neuropeptide chain, whether anger or love, dependent on the exact sequence and composition of these links. Imagine, every sensation or emotion one has ever experienced, depending upon the makeup of these short neuropeptide chains, like popcorn on a string, carrying our behavioral destiny. These linked peptides are then packaged into transport vesicles that are shuttled across the cytoplasm to the Golgi apparatus. The operation of the Golgi apparatus, this marvel of complexity, which only recently has begun to reveal its secrets to research scientists, has been likened to that of a post office. Electron microscopy has revealed that its general structure is comparable to a stack of "letters" shaped like hotcakes and bound by a common membrane. It is here that vesicles of proteins are linked with certain sugars, zip-code fashion, and directed to their final destination within and without the cell, and it is here that the dolichols play their unique role. In the absence of sufficient dolichol this delicate process cannot properly take place.

Most of us are familiar with the blocking action of statins on ubiquinone but few really understand the consequence of dolichol suppression by statin drug use. When I was in medical school, dolichols and neuropeptides were unknown or much too vague a concept to talk about. Few physicians readily comprehend what has been learned in the past few decades without having done detailed study of journals of biochemistry and molecular biology, so few practicing physicians will find this material familiar. Without sufficient dolichols, the intricate process of neuropeptide formation and transport cannot occur. Intracellular chaos can result, as various proteins are not directed to their proper target and are, in effect, dead-lettered. The post office analogy, though childishly simple, comes very close to describing the Golgi apparatus function as we understand it today and the entire process is orchestrated by dolichols.

There is no disputing either statins' inhibition of dolichol synthesis or dolichol's vital role in neuropeptide formation. Since our neuropeptides are involved in so many areas of physiology, possible manifestations of impaired neuropeptide function are protean, suggesting that even the most obscure of patient symptoms may be associated with statin use. Researchers in this field are reporting the frequent association of statin use with such symptoms as hostility, aggressiveness, irritability, homicidal actions, road rage type behavior, exacerbation of alcohol and drug addiction, proneness to depression, suicidal thoughts, failed suicidal attempts and occasional suicide successes[6]. Such behavioral manifestations are felt to be related to dolichol inhibition and altered neuropeptide formation.

The following are just a few of the many case reports I have received from people who report emotional and behavioral side effects associated with their use of statin drugs:

"I saw your article on the internet. My father who is 70 years, about 3 months ago started having pressure on the right side of his head and nervousness - he feels like he is losing his mind - he says it feels like something is crawling inside his legs - he is miserable. His primary care physician says it is depression and increased his Zoloft - that has been 2 weeks ago - and he is no better. He says his mind just won't let him think - and everything seems confusing to him. I tried to talk with the physician about the Lipitor that he has been taking for years - because I saw on the internet that Lipitor could cause problems with patients who were also on Lanoxin (it said it could build up a toxin). Do you know anything that might help us? The physician won't have it any other way but depression - I just don't see that - my father has never been depressed a day in his life."

I read your website with much interest, and also hope. My mother has struggled with high cholesterol for many years, specifically with her triglyceride levels. Diet did not alter her levels. I may add that she is an active 66-year who walks 4 miles a day, and is in great physical shape. About 9 months ago, my siblings and I noticed that she did not call us as much, and that when we talked with her by phone or in person, she seemed to not recall past conversations or details. She has gotten worse, where she seems withdrawn from conversations, and uninterested in things that happen around her. This is not all of the time, as sometimes she seems like her old self. She is a recently retired RN who worked for 30 years in the field. She is currently taking Lipitor and Pravachol to control the cholesterol, and has been put on a mild dose of medication to stimulate the brain (unsure of its name, but is used to treat early signs of dementia). I have produced two articles from the Wall Street Journal regarding the statin drugs and the effective on memory for my dad who has taken them to the physician. He was told that they are a top-notch treatment center, which none of us denies, and that statin drugs do not affect the memory. That being said in a very long explanation, do you have any suggestions? My obvious first thought is to seek another opinion, and to take her off of the statins to see if this makes a difference. If the memory loss is caused by the Lipitor, then we can deal with that, but if it is the beginnings of something more serious, then a different approach to my siblings and I would be in order to take advantage of her now. Thank you. Your site has allowed me to see that we can't take no for an answer about getting her off of Lipitor. I hope it inspires others to check into things a bit further."

"I hope you can help me. My husband was on Lipitor for at least 3 years, and suddenly he lost his ability to speak. During this time he was on a low fat diet and lost 42 pounds, however, no one ever mentioned taking him off this poison drug. Now he is unable to function and they, the head doctors, say he is psychotic. A good man with an excellent job, dealing with very detailed work, is now unable to function. True, he has had some emotional problems, he had a falling out with a son, and now he cannot see his grandchildren. Suddenly he lost his ability to speak, well not suddenly but over a six-month period."

CHAPTER 5
Statins and NF-kB

Even if the dedicated researchers of the pharmaceutical industry discover a way around the side effect mechanisms already described, even greater hurdles exist from our recent evidence that statins work not by cholesterol manipulation but by some basic anti-inflammatory mechanism.

Key to this is a substance known as nuclear factor kappa B. All statins inhibit this vital step in our immune system's ability to defend us from alien forces[1]. Whether by being the recipient of a donor kidney or under attack by bacteria or viruses, our immune system has evolved a defensive strategy in which suppression of inflammation, triggered by nuclear factor kappa B, plays a vital role[2]. Such stimulants to inflammation include the foreign by-products of arterial inflammation and damage. Statin drugs are known to suppress this nuclear factor kappa B (NF-kB) response and thereby open a completely novel opportunity for, unpredictable and potentially disastrous consequences.

At best, our HMG Co-A reductase inhibitors are blunt instruments and our immuno-defense system is both delicate and complex. During eons of co-existence of our complex multicellular life forms with competing, simpler unicellular organisms, there have developed many different forms of defensive and offensive strategy - all dealing with the needs of one or the other of these dueling organisms to gain a survival advantage[3,4,5]. We have had 3.5 billion years to work out our defense systems against widely diverse challenges and NF-kB is key to all of them. If we thought the complexity of cholesterol manufacture by our body is complex, it is child's play compared to what is involved in anti-infection and immuno-modulation. Now, throw in a statin and try to predict the consequences.

NF-kB in its several forms is known to molecular biologists as a transcription factor and my bringing more than a smattering of this complex subject to your attention would risk losing you from terminal boredom, so skim the following very lightly. I warned you this is challenging - how could a history of a 3.5 billion year war be otherwise? NF-kB resides in the cytoplasm of each cell in five different forms known to our molecular biologists as family. The offspring of these family members, known as dimers, remain firmly held in check in the cytoplasm by certain inhibitory proteins until a release signal is received, allowing our now activated NF-kB to enter the nucleus of the cell. It is there, in the nucleus, that it completes its mission in life to stimulate genes and manufacture proteins necessary for such diverse tasks as monocyte adhesion, macrophage recruitment, smooth muscle migration and platelet activation, key elements of our defensive inflammatory response.

With so many steps involved, a good strategist could predict many different forms of assault by dedicated viruses, bacteria and other forms of single celled life, for this war is basically that of the monocellular rulers originally dominating life on our planet against we multicellular usurpers. Therefore it should come as no surprise that some of these defenders have managed to gain an advantage over us, their adversary, by inhibiting NF-kB while others succeed by enhancing NF-kB[6,7,8,9]. Others manage both sides of the coin. E. coli, one of our most common infectious agents, prevents NF-kB from entering the nucleus, thereby enabling this ubiquitous organism freer access to our bladder walls and urethras. Through a similar process of checkmate, another common bacteria, Salmonella, inhibits our anti-inflammatory response sufficiently long to allow bacterial colonization of the lining of the gut, giving a decided advantage to "their" side. On the other hand, some Chlamydia organisms, warring against the urogenital systems of both men and women, have evolved a distinct advantage by enhancing our NF-kB, thereby assuring increased survival of infected cells in our urinary and reproductive systems. On a far more serious note, the very common Epstein-Barr virus causing infectious mononucleosis uses NF-kB inhibition to help destroy our protective "T " cells as part of our common teenage "mono" presentation but when it decides to go on a malignant rampage, triggering nasopharyngeal carcinoma and Burkitt's lymphoma, it does so through sustained NF-kB activation. The list goes on and on with other microorganisms and foreign antigens of all kinds, numbering thousands of variations of these basic themes.

So now let us return to statin drugs and their now well-established effect of inhibition of NF-kB. What does this really mean in our ancient struggle with disease organisms and our immune system's competence? It means while taking statins we are likely to be far more susceptible to certain common infectious agents but at the same time may be somewhat more resistant to others. In the case of the Epstein Barr virus, perhaps we will see more " mono" but, fortunately, less nasopharyngeal carcinoma and Burkitt's lymphoma. But the reality is that we do not as yet know because this new statin role of NF-kB inhibition has only just been recognized. The potential for increased risk of both infectious disease and malignancy is there, for both depend upon our immune system's competence. Tossing the statin sledgehammer into this system is perhaps quite comparable in effect to the rampages of "a bull in a china shop" and it is far too soon to tell about most malignant changes. The implications of the very recent drug company promotion of statin drugs for organ transplant recipients and as adjunctive therapy in the treatment of auto-immune diseases[10,11] are sobering, indeed, for these drugs can only work in this capacity at the risk of causing mischief elsewhere. One must admire the drug companies' ability for "positive spin" on a very alarming proposition, or is it arrogance? One cannot have the one without the other. The sense of cynicism here is overwhelming to me.

Increased cancer deaths among recipients of statin drugs already are being observed. Ravnskov in his, The Cholesterol Myths, has reported from the recent PROSPER trial[12] that statin therapy increased the incidence of cancer deaths, completely offsetting the slight decrease in deaths from cardiovascular disease. As Dr. Paul Rosch predicted in his Weston Price Foundation presentation of May 2003[13], the Japan Lipid Intervention trial[14] observed excess deaths from malignancy in their so-called statin "hyper-responder" group. Of the 12 cancer deaths reported in this group, whose cholesterol's plummeted deeply with statin use, four were from gastric cancer and two were from lung cancer. Although other factors may have played a role, this heightened cancer risk may well be based on at least partial loss of immuno-resistance secondary to NF-kB inhibition.

How strange it is that a class of drugs developed solely for the purpose to interfering with the biosynthesis of cholesterol has now been shown to reduce cardiovascular risk by an anti-inflammatory role completely unrelated to cholesterol manipulation. Generally speaking this should by a welcome observation, for atherosclerosis with all of its consequences is based primarily upon inflammation within the arterial walls. Now, however, any optimism we might have had is thoroughly tempered by our growing realization that a statin's effect is based upon interference with our most basic immuno defense system. The potential consequences are frightening.

CHAPTER 6
The Role of Cholesterol in the Body

There is no doubt that the present notoriety of cholesterol has all but obscured its physiological importance and necessity in our bodies. Cholesterol is not only the most common organic molecule in our brain; it is also distributed intimately throughout our entire body. It is an essential constituent of the membrane surrounding every cell. The presence of cholesterol in this fatty double layer of the cell wall adjusts the fluidity and rigidity of this membrane to the proper value for both cell stability and function.

Additionally, cholesterol is the precursor for a whole class of hormones known as the steroid hormones that are absolutely critical for life, as we know it. These hormones determine our sexuality, control the reproductive process, and regulate blood sugar levels and mineral metabolism. This same substance that society has been taught to fear happens to be our sole source for androgen, estrogen and progesterone. Researchers marvel at the remarkable similarity in chemical structure these sex hormones have with each other and with the original cholesterol parent from which they are derived. One might say the glaring family resemblance attests to the mighty power of a methyl group here and a carboxyl group there. The destiny of us all is marvelously controlled by such seemingly minor changes.

This same notorious cholesterol substance is also the parent of a pair of steroid hormones called aldosterone and cortisol[1]. Aldosterone protects the body from excessive loss of sodium and water and is known in scientific circles as a mineralocorticoid. It is absolutely vital for life. Without an adequate supply of aldosterone we would be like an ill-prepared desert traveler destined to die of thirst and dehydration under the glaring rays of a merciless sun as water and salt escape from his body.

Cortisol is known as a glucocorticoid because it helps control blood sugar levels and glucose metabolism, but it also has powerful mineralocorticoid and immune system functions and is fundamentally involved in the biologic response to the stress in our lives.

Both of these vital substances are created in the cortex, the outer shell of the adrenal glands. When the adrenal cortex is destroyed by accident, surgery or disease, death occurs within days unless the patient receives aldosterone and cortisol. Like the sex hormones mentioned above, there can be no aldosterone or cortisol unless an adequate supply of the parent substance, cholesterol, is available. So much of our life is dependent on this remarkable substance.

And where would we be without calcitrol[2]? Another offspring of cholesterol, this remarkable steroid hormone is charged with the responsibility for maintaining the proper level of calcium in our bodies. Like sodium, serum calcium must be maintained by the body within a very narrow range for us to function. Without calcitrol the calcium we ingest would pass through our bowels unclaimed.

The calcium in our teeth and bones would diminish rapidly, leading to advanced osteoporosis, skeletal weakness and fractures. Without calcium, nerve transmission to our muscles would fail, resulting in a hyperexcitable state. We have all seen cartoons and movies where a doctor gets an exaggerated knee jerk response while checking a patient's reflexes, a sure sign of low calcium levels. Very low calcium levels result in massive seizures of muscles, incompatible with life, in a condition known as generalized tetany. Such is the power of a simple element like calcium on our bodies if homeostatic levels are violated. Proper levels of serum calcium are also vital for optimum function of our immune systems.

Again, cholesterol is the basis of all these steroid hormones without which life, as we know it, would not be possible. But, by no means is the list of cholesterol's contributions to body function exhausted, for there is another class of cholesterol's steroid offspring without which our metabolic well-being might be in serious jeopardy: the production of bile acids. Secreted by the liver and stored in the gall bladder, bile makes it possible for us to emulsify fats and other nutrients. Without bile, we could not digest and absorb the fats in our diet. In the absence of sufficient bile acids we would all be like those unfortunate souls whose intestinal villi are rudimentary or deficient, which causes them to produce voluminous stools of undigested material while they slowly starve.

The pharmaceutical industry would lead us to believe that rapidly bottoming out our natural cholesterol levels through the use of their highly touted statin drugs is a relatively innocuous process of definite benefit to society. But as we learn more each day of this ubiquitous and unique substance, we must question the veracity of their medical advisors. Cholesterol is perhaps the most important substance in our lives for we could not live without an abundant supply of it in our bodies. Researchers everywhere are learning how extraordinarily complex and often surprising are the pathways that produce and metabolize cholesterol in our bodies. Admittedly, even after decades of study of this remarkable chemical, we still have much to learn.

Pfreiger's announcement on 9 November 2001 about the discovery of the identity of the elusive synaptogenic factor responsible for the development of synapses, the highly specialized contact sites between adjacent neurons in the brain, deserves to be cited again in the context of cholesterol's vast importance to our bodies[3]. Neuronal transmission, the very essence of who we are, is absolutely dependent upon abundant cholesterol reserves. The synaptogenic factor was shown to be the notorious substance cholesterol!

The so-called glial cells, the non-nervous or supporting tissue of the brain and spinal cord long suspected of providing certain housekeeping functions, were shown to produce their own supply of cholesterol for the specific purpose of providing nerve cells with this vital synaptic component.

This should be sobering news for those in the pharmaceutical industry developing drugs which interfere with cholesterol synthesis, the mechanism of action of all our statins. One wonders how anyone knowing the mechanism of brain cholesterol synthesis by our glial cells can seriously challenge the reality of cognitive side effects from statin drug use. The only surprise is that there are not more reported cases of memory impairment, amnesia, confusion and disorientation.

This is heady stuff, indeed, for a substance with such bad press. When and if the industry finally vindicates cholesterol, it will not be unlike posthumously elevating Al Capone to knighthood.

This discussion of the biological importance of cholesterol would not be complete without a review of recent research information concerning some of the other more sobering implications of excessively low serum cholesterol concentrations in our bodies.

Despite Muldoon's findings of no increase in suicides, accidents and violence in his cholesterol lowering treatment groups[5], Golomb reported a significant association between low or lowered cholesterol levels and violence across many types of studies[6]. As principal investigator of the National Institutes of Health funded study at University of California San Diego, College of Medicine, Dr. Golomb is the recipient of thousands of patient case reports on statin drug side effects.

Whereas Wolozin, et al, reported decreased prevalence of dementia associated with statin drug use[7], Golomb countered in a letter to the editor of Archives of Neurology[8] that the Wolozin data could be taken to support a contrary conclusion--that high cholesterol protects against dementia. Golomb cited her many reports from statin users reporting cognitive loss frequently requiring medical work-ups for Alzheimer's disease and implying that the lowered cholesterol levels in such patients appeared to be a contributing factor. Her work is supported by Pfreiger's recent observation that Alzheimer's disease is characterized by a progressive and irreversible loss of neurons and synapses associated with cholesterol deficit[9]. Additionally, Henry Lorin, in his new book, Alzheimer's Solved, has stressed the critical role of low cholesterol in the development of Alzheimer's disease[10]. In light of this one can only shake his head in wonder at the many studies planned or actually under way purporting to prove statins' benefit for this tragic condition.

That low or lowered cholesterol also contributes to aggressive behavior, violence, depression, and mood disturbance has led Kaplan at Yale University's School of Medicine and others to propose a cholesterol/serotonin hypothesis to explain the relationship[11,12,13,14,15]. Buydens-Branchey reported a strong relationship of low plasma levels of cholesterol and relapse in cocaine addicts[16]. Although the authors did not report specifically on the effect of cholesterol lowering medication on their patients, the inference is inescapable that such medication, especially with the statin class of drugs, might seriously aggravate the addiction problem.

As if the preceding were not sufficiently sobering concerning the hazards of low or lowered serum cholesterol, we have the report of Horwich et al[17], that low cholesterol is a strong, independent predictor of impaired survival in older heart failure patients. From the work of Peter Langsjoen, we suspect a major contribution of coenzyme Q10 deficiency in these cases if such patients were on statins, but the authors caution that they did not have data on the patients' medical regimens. They imply, however, that low serum cholesterol is an independent marker of increased mortality in their patient group, suggesting mechanisms other than statin-induced ubiquinone deficiency.

Like many other, if not all, chemical constituents of our bodies, there may well be an ideal level of cholesterol in each of us. Low or lowered cholesterol - below our presumed ideal, "normal" range, and DNA mandated to be different in each of us, seems to be associated with a wide-ranging spectrum of problems from memory impairment, depression, suicide and dementia, to drug addiction relapse, and even with heart failure in our elderly. These observations are thoroughly documented and deserve thoughtful consideration by physicians prescribing statin drugs.

We will present more on the misguided war on cholesterol in the groundbreaking research of Dr. Kilmer McCully[18], who further defines the innocence of natural cholesterol in favor of the culpability of homocysteine in the causation of cardiovascular disease as he points his finger at the true problem of atherosclerosis and scourge of strokes and heart attacks – inflammation!

Chapter 7
Role of Inflammation in Atherosclerosis

No one has done more or worked harder in the past 35 years to determine the cause of arteriosclerosis than Dr. Kilmer McCully[1]. His persistent, pioneering research has revealed a wealth of knowledge about the process of this disease, our most common cause of premature death. Ignoring the huge tide of contrary medical opinion during that period, he insisted that there was more to the etiology of arteriosclerosis than high serum cholesterol. And he was correct, as this chapter will show. Had the medical research field been receptive to his findings or even willing to consider causes other than cholesterol, the present flood of prescriptions for cholesterol-lowering statin drugs with their devastating side effects might never have occurred.

He had discovered that cholesterol comes in several different varieties. Some, known as oxycholesterol, contain extra oxygen atoms. Whereas pure cholesterol, free of all traces of oxycholesterol, is innocuous when injected into the arteries of experimental animals, oxycholesterol, obtained simply by exposing cholesterol to oxygen, becomes toxic and highly effective in producing arteriosclerosis in animals. Inflammation caused by this toxic agent could easily trigger a reaction resulting in elevated CRP. Natural cholesterol is innocuous. Oxycholesterol causes intense inflammation but this is not the end of the story.

Now McCully had the reason why animals fed cholesterol in their feed got atherosclerosis but what about the results of autopsies done on Korean and Vietnam casualties? Most doctors were astonished to learn that the arteries of these 18 to 22-year old young men were laced with lipid streaks, foam cells and atheromatous plaques. Our story is now just beginning!

The country was now about to embark on a three decade long application of the cholesterol/fat approach for the control of heart disease. Powered by ample federal funding, the bandwagon began to roll, carrying politicians, university administrators and directors of health departments and health agencies in its wake. These were the days of the Heart Disease, Cancer and Stroke legislation, which suddenly put universities into the health-care-delivery loop where a major effort was the promotion of cholesterol-control programs at the community levels.

As physicians we began to write more and more prescriptions for cholesterol-lowering drugs. We lectured at service clubs and even to school groups on the benefit of cholesterol control and a fat-restricted diet. Any doctor not marching in this parade was considered academically deficient. Thoroughly endorsed by the medical and pharmaceutical establishments, cholesterol control drugs seemed to be the answer. These early drugs had side effects that were at times serious and even disabling, but the statin drugs were yet to be discovered and we encountered no amnesia, forgetfulness, confusion or disorientation.

Fortunately, not everyone accepted the cholesterol theory. Kilmer McCully, MD, working at Harvard during the late 60s, had been involved in research that suggested a role for factors other than cholesterol and LDL in the etiology of arteriosclerosis. This was an almost inconceivable thought in those days. His interest was aroused when, as a member of the Harvard human genetics group, he was present when pediatricians presented the story of the death of an eight-year old boy, suffering from a disease called homocysteinuria. The child had died of a stroke at that tender age.

This rare condition had been discovered only six years earlier by medical investigators in Belfast. In the ensuing years, several more cases were identified. In this condition, a genetic error occurs in a liver enzyme known as cystathionine synthase. When this happens, the amino acid, homocysteine, derived from the normal breakdown of protein in the diet, cannot be metabolized by the liver as usual and builds up to toxic levels. The arteries in these cases are abnormal, with hardening and loss of elasticity that greatly increase the tendency for heart attacks and strokes. Not only did McCully focus on this observation, but he also knew of the work of George Spaeth, an ophthalmologist friend, who informed him of the dramatically beneficial effect of vitamin B6 supplementation on some of the homocysteinuria patients he had treated. Spaeth's homocysteinuria patients often suffered from a dislocated lens. He reported his observation to McCully that the excretion of homocysteine in the urine of such patients frequently could be increased dramatically by vitamin B6. Two seeds were firmly planted in Kilmer McCully's receptive mind: the amino acid homocysteine, if elevated, causes a condition remarkably like arteriosclerosis; and a simple vitamin, B6, could lower homocysteine levels. He was elated with this hint that a nutritional factor other than cholesterol might be involved, but his thinking was nothing more than a tiny candle lighting the darkness of lack of knowledge of this disease. He was alone with his concept and his original ideas fell on ears deafened by the roar of the cholesterol juggernaut.

McCully hurried to his laboratory and began to apply his skills as a pathologist to some of the original material from the homocysteinuria case discussed at the genetics meeting. He found some paraffin blocks containing tissue from the young boy and a few of the original slides. Soon he was able to confirm that, indeed, the walls of the carotid arteries leading to the brain were severely thickened and damaged by arteriosclerosis, a form of hardening of the arteries. He now knew this disastrous blood vessel disease had caused the stroke that had killed the young boy. He found scattered, widespread changes in virtually all the small arteries of the body. He found neither cholesterol deposits nor plaques, just the routine calcified sclerosis and narrowing that he had come to associate with arteriosclerosis of the elderly.

Soon he had identified ten more cases of homocysteinuria in children, many of whom, had died of blood clots to the brain, heart and kidneys. All showed the hardening of the arteries and loss of elasticity associated with fibrous plaques. An abnormal reactivity of the blood platelets was evident in these patients, which accounted for the tendency toward formation of blood clots. Somehow, the presence of elevated homocysteine in the blood had caused the blood platelets to cluster more readily.

Some time later at another genetics conference, McCully learned of another homocystinuria-like case: a two-month-old baby that had died despite aggressive attempts at therapy. This time, the urine contained both homocysteine and another substance called cystathionine, also related to homocysteine. In the case of this unfortunate baby, its metabolic passageway was deficient in a different enzyme and the conversion would have required vitamin B12. When McCully examined the slides of the baby's arteries he found the same arteriosclerosis changes noted in all the previous cases.

By now one should call McCully a medical detective, for that is what he had become. He admits he had difficulty sleeping for several weeks after this discovery because he knew he was on to something of extreme importance.

Like many scientists before him McCully had doubted the cholesterol hypothesis because cholesterol makes up so much of the human body and is so intimately involved in metabolism and physiology. And cholesterol is a major component of the human brain. How could such a substance be sufficiently toxic to cause arterial damage? It did not make any sense to him.

Meanwhile it was now 1970 and researchers directed their attention to LDL in its Jekyll and Hyde guise, trying to understand why this innocuous substance behaved so erratically. In one instance it would provoke strong macrophage response leading to foam cell production, and at another time or in another form, its monocyte macrophages caused no pathological response.

McCully thought it likely that the receptor for LDL on the membranes of the endothelial cells lining the arteries was the determining factor and that the "activated" LDL, the process that makes LDL extremely "tasty" to a wandering monocyte, somehow takes place in these same cells. One wonders if this just might be where the lipoprotein (a) of Pauling and Rath[2] fits into the picture. First reported in 1991, this cholesterol carrying substance, so vital to arterial repair, had been routinely mistaken for regular LDL before then. The jury is still out on this idea, but research evidence is accumulating.

McCully lacked enthusiasm for the cholesterol/fat hypothesis prevalent in most of his co-workers. Not only was he drawn by the common sense appeal of his research-proven protein toxicity/vitamin deficiency theory, but he also knew the cholesterol hypothesis was lacking in several major respects. The most glaring deficiency of the then current cholesterol/fat hypothesis, according to McCully, was the fact that "the majority of patients with coronary heart disease, stroke and other forms of arteriosclerotic disease have no evidence of elevated cholesterol or LDL levels[3].

McCully reported in his 1990 study[4] of 194 consecutive autopsy studies of mostly male veterans of finding only 8 percent of cases with severe arteriosclerosis that had total cholesterol levels greater than 250 mg/dL. He found the average blood cholesterol in the group with the severest disease was 186 mg/dL. This observation, perhaps more than any other, convinced McCully that medical researchers had to look elsewhere. The cholesterol/fat hypothesis provided no answers for this prevalent observation nor did it offer any reasonable explanation for how so ubiquitous a substance as cholesterol, a major and vital component of the human body, could provoke the onset of arteriosclerosis.

Another glaring deficiency of the cholesterol/fat etiology for arteriosclerosis was the observation, mentioned previously, from autopsies done on Korea and Vietnam military casualties. When one thinks about it, how could the extensive lipid streaks and early arteriosclerosis present in so many of these young men, many still in their teens, be attributable to a cholesterol causation when cholesterol/LDL levels in the young, supremely conditioned group were "rock bottom low?"

McCully had few allies during this time. Practicing physicians had a mindset created by decades of cholesterol/fat "brainwashing". The pharmaceutical industry had concentrated for decades on the development of ever more effective cholesterol control drugs. To say the endeavor was lucrative is a masterpiece of understatement. Billions of dollars yearly are involved; the profits are almost shameful in their excess. So the bandwagon had turned into a "cash cow" for the pharmaceutical industry and there were no friends for Dr. McCully there. Even the food industry would turn up its nose at a man who threatened their highly profitable, low cholesterol, processed foods and unsaturated oils by suggesting that relatively unprofitable fresh produce and, of all things, vitamin supplementation are healthy substitutes.

Finally, after "baiting the administrative lion for years" by investigating "dark alleys" and despite his 28-year affiliation, McCully's staff appointment ended December 31, 1978. One can only applaud the conviction of this man who, despite this setback, persevered. Gradually, as if to help McCully emerge from his doldrums, the seeds of a homocysteine causation of arteriosclerosis began to germinate and emerge from the research establishment.

Bridget and David Wilcken[5] began to publish their series of papers devoted to the study of homocysteine's role in heart disease. These doctors found that methionine given to patients with established heart disease resulted in large increases in serum homocysteine.

Many other epidemiological studies followed over the next two decades comparing the homocysteine levels of patients with heart disease, stroke, peripheral vascular disease, kidney failure, and even deep vein thrombophlebitis, with the blood homocysteine levels of normal controls. The current result of these studies is a consensus among medical investigators such as Boushey[6] that elevation of blood homocysteine levels is a strong independent risk factor for the development of arteriosclerotic disease.

The list of studies vindicating McCully's departure from established research pathways now goes on and on. Clearly, Kilmer McCully was "on to something" back at Harvard when he was denied continued affiliation with their "forward thinking" research institution because "he had failed to prove his theory."

After years of study, the role of cholesterol in atheroma formation must be viewed as a passive one. There is now little doubt that a major cause of arteriosclerosis is the methionine/homocysteine metabolic interplay but other factors are likely to be involved. Even McCully will admit that adding together the possible contributions of hereditary predisposition, and even the most pessimistic estimate of dietary deficiencies of folic acid and vitamins B6 and B12 in the general public will not explain more than 40% of cardiovascular disease. Other researchers postulate that trans fats, grossly abnormal omega-3/omega-6 ratio, magnesium deficiency, inherent thrombotic tendencies, and even subtle anti-oxidant deficiencies, as possible contributing factors. Kauffman wrote an excellent review of this subject in 2000[7].

Despite the glowing reports in the press, strong evidence exists that cholesterol levels do not matter. Ravnskov[8] summarizes that statin drug therapy is reported to be almost as effective for high risk women as for men, despite the fact that most studies have shown that cholesterol is not a risk factor for women. Additionally, the elderly with high risk are protected just as much as younger individuals, although all studies have shown that high cholesterol is only a weak factor for men older than fifty. Another observation mitigating against a cholesterol explanation for statin effectiveness is the consistent finding that strokes are reduced after statin therapy, even though high cholesterol is only a weak risk factor for stroke. Further confounding a possible cholesterol effect mechanism for statins is the fact that they protect regardless of whether the patient's cholesterol is high or low.

For these reasons cholesterol can no longer be cited as the sole cause of any patient's progressive arteriosclerosis any more than can smoking, hypertension, obesity or diabetes. It must be considered just another risk factor deserving attention. All of our present well-intentioned attempts at controlling cholesterol do little for the underlying arteriosclerosis or tendency for strokes and heart attacks.

So McCully has made a strong case for inflammation not cholesterol to be the culprit in cardiovascular disease and introduced the possibility that nutritional factors other than cholesterol are involved. There is now a compelling reason for radical change in our nation's diet and less dependence on pharmaceutical "crutches". To fight arteriosclerosis one must fight its cause. We need nutrition and health programs directed at such causes of inflammation as McCully's homocysteine, omega-3 deficiency and other arterial damaging factors that his research has led us to - the true causes of arteriosclerosis. Only in this way will we decrease our dependence on the statin class of drugs with their mind-robbing potential. We insist that transient global amnesia, permanent neuromuscular debility and profound behavioral changes are not acceptable drug side effects! But we must not lose sight of the fact that despite their many shortcomings, our statins remain powerful anti-inflammatory agents and inflammation has is now the culprit. One might ask why we still are using cholesterol-lowering doses of statins when recent research points at inflammation not cholesterol as the real problem? I will return to this important consideration in subsequent chapters.

CHAPTER 8
Our Misguided War on Cholesterol

A major part of our heart attack and stroke prevention efforts these past several decades has been the so-called cholesterol-modified, low-fat diet. During this time our morbidity and mortality from arteriosclerosis has changed little, if at all. True, through high-tech surgical intervention we have accomplished a miracle of restoring blood to threatened or damaged organs, but the prevalence of progressive arterial blockage remains largely unchanged. Apparently we have done nothing to stop or even slow down this dreaded condition. Our burgeoning statin drug industry now feeds on nearly fifty million users and still, they say, we are not reaching all the people who should be on it. Some would call this medical progress but I must call it medical failure!

"If the members of the American medical establishment were to have a collective find-yourself-standing-naked-in-Times-Square-type nightmare, this might be it. They spend 30 years ridiculing Robert Atkins, author of the phenomenally best selling, Dr. Atkins' New Diet Revolution[1], accusing the author of quackery and fraud, only to discover that the unrepentant Atkins was right all along. Or maybe it's this: they find that their very own dietary recommendations - eat less fat and more carbohydrates - are the cause of the rampaging epidemic of obesity in America. Or, just possibly this: they find out both of the above are true." This quote is from Gary Taubes' very perceptive New York Times article, "What If It's All Been a Big Fat Lie[2]?" and who among us, aware of the severity of the weight problems in this country, cannot applaud another avenue of inquiry into its cause?

In 1972, just as the American Medical Association and the American Heart Association started the low cholesterol/low fat juggernaut on its fateful advance through the American public, a then little-known doctor by the name of Robert Atkins started his own trajectory, named Diet Revolution. He managed to sell millions of copies of his book by promising that a diet completely contradictory to the medical establishment recommendations was the way to go. He promised the public they would lose weight by eating steak, eggs and butter to their heart's desire because fat was harmless. It was the carbohydrates--the pasta, rice, bagels and sugar-- that caused obesity and heart disease, he contended. Atkins popularized his high-fat diet to such an extent that the American Medical Association considered his book and philosophy a threat to public health. Because of AMA pressure, Atkins was forced to defend his diet in congressional hearings.

The thrust of Atkin's diet and of the many similar carbohydrate restrictive diets that followed, of course, was to partake of foodstuffs requiring minimal insulin secretion, thereby tending to stabilize the hunger mechanism.

Since Atkins' debut in 1972, additional best selling diet books including Protein Power[3], The Zone[4], Sugar Busters[5], Kilmer McCully's The Heart Revolution[6], and others have polarized the American public on the subject of weight by recommending minor variations on the low carbohydrate/ liberal fat theme. All of them run contrary to the low cholesterol/low fat theme of organized medicine. The AMA preached that obesity and heart disease are caused by the excessive consumption of fat; the best sellers preached that carbohydrate is the villain and that fat is harmless. Despite the popularity of such books, the impact of organized medicine and the combined effects of our pharmaceutical and food industries have been far greater on the American public, and on all kinds of institutional food.

The result is our present obesity epidemic, our worsening incidence of Type 2 diabetes, and the realization that despite lowering blood cholesterols, our incidence of arteriosclerosis and heart disease differs very little, if at all, from thirty years ago. Some are finally ready to say the low cholesterol/modified fat diet has been an unhappy failure on the part of organized medicine.

Adding to this very real confusion, stirring the pot of conflicting ideology, so to speak, is the rapidly evolving reality that the notorious cholesterol may not be Public Enemy No.1, after all. Kilmer McCully's proposition that arteriosclerosis is largely an inflammatory response due to alteration in the homocysteine/methionine metabolic pathways with cholesterol assuming a passive role, at best, is rapidly gaining support. Although the jury still is out on this proposition, it begins to seem very likely that the medical establishment, fifty years ago, may have put all its many prestigious eggs in the wrong basket. If you want to go after arteriosclerosis, place your sights on inflammation from homocysteine toxicity and nutritional deficiencies, not cholesterol! It seems impossible to believe that we have been wrong for all this time but it is true.

Walter Willett, Chairman of the Department of Nutrition at the Harvard School of Public Health in Boston, reports from his comprehensive diet and health study[7], the largest yet, that his preliminary data clearly contradict the low cholesterol/low fat ideology. In an ABC interview on 21 November 2002, Dr. Willett stated, "The public has been told for many years that fats are bad and carbohydrates are good." This radical departure from current nutritional philosophy literally turns USDA's food pyramid on its head. One can imagine the reaction of tens of thousands of well meaning dietitians and nutritionists to such heresy. To make matters even worse he added, "In fact, we've known for 30 or 40 years that that's not really true." Why, one might ask, was this respected and hallowed institution unable to muscle this information into national policy? Not only has our present nutritional philosophy failed to prevent coronary artery disease and ischemic stroke incidence but it also seems to have contributed directly to our obesity epidemic.

Next door, at Harvard's pediatric obesity clinic, David Ludwig stresses the negative impact of carbohydrates on insulin, blood sugar, fat metabolism and appetite - basic endocrinology apparently not fully appreciated thirty years earlier. To eat more fat-free carbohydrates inevitably leads to hunger and indulgence, then weight gain.

"For a large percentage of the population, low-fat diets are counter-productive," Taubes reports from his interview with the director of obesity research at Harvard's Joslin Diabetes Center. "They have the paradoxical effect of making people gain weight."

How is it possible that a country like ours has arrived at such a point where doctors who can find the time to consider and ponder such matters are beginning to feel uncomfortable and more than a little ashamed?

As Sally Fallon and Mary G. Enig have reported in their perceptive article, "The Mediterranean Diet - Pasta or Pastrami[8]?" it was Ancel Keys, then visiting professor at Oxford in 1951, who first took note of the apparent benefits of the Italian national diet. He claimed this diet was characterized by abundant plant foods, fresh fruits and grains. As Professor Gino Bergami, Professor of Physiology at the University of Naples, reported to him at the first conference of the United Nation's Food and Agriculture Organization in Rome, "coronary heart disease was no problem in Naples."

Dr. Keys was intrigued with this comment and, shortly thereafter, he and his wife departed from their 1952 unheated apartment and the food rations of England to live for a while in sunny Naples. There, as a team, they studied this classic Italian diet but incorrectly deducing that it was low in fat, especially saturated fat. Serum cholesterol measurements of the local citizens seemed to confirm the apparent benefits. They concluded there was an association between diet, serum cholesterol and coronary heart disease[9].

As Fallon and Enig reported, at first, Dr. Keys found little support for his revolutionary theories. But he encountered a sympathetic listener in 1952 when he presented his views to a small audience in New York at Mt. Sinai Hospital. Fred Epstein, convinced by Keys' data, began spreading the message "with great effect" over Europe and America. Keys expanded his studies and later, in 1970, published his Seven Countries Study[10], in which it was later found that he had used selective data[11].

After this research was published, the "Keys' diet" became government policy and the darling of both the American Medical Association and the American Heart Association. This was the well-documented and perhaps poorly defined origin of America's modified fat/low cholesterol rationale for national diet, which dominated scientific thinking and research for the next thirty years. Since that time unfortunate changes have occurred in the so-called Mediterranean diet. The food now served commonly is far from the former Mediterranean pattern. As Fallon and Enig so colorfully describe,

"It must be distressing (for Keys) to observe sophisticated Italians feasting on such travesties as pasta Alfredo, veal scaloppini and prosciutto, especially to one who had taken the stringent vows of the diet priesthood." Study after study now finds the so - called Keys' Mediterranean diet largely a myth - probably a temporary result of the aftermath of World War II deprivation and half a decade of social conflict but one that became the basis of our low cholesterol/low fat diet.

Once our National Institutes of Health had signed off on the concept, however, the American food industry - suspected by some to be behind the whole thing - quickly joined in with a never-ending parade of reduced fat products to meet the new recommendations. The fat content, which to a great extent gives processed food much of its flavor, was eliminated from many cookies and chips, ice cream, milk, cheese and yogurt and replaced by carbohydrates. These carbohydrates were inevitably the refined variety, relying heavily on refined sugar or starch, which, though adding bulk and perhaps taste, resulted in the public eating almost pure sugar, metabolically speaking. Aided and abetted by the missionary zeal of well-intentioned dietitians, health organizations, consumer groups and even cookbook writers, one could almost see America's waistlines expanding.

The impact of low fat/high carbohydrate diets on serum triglycerides was and is potentially lethal. By the late 1960s, triglyceride levels were already rising, protective HDL levels were falling and Type

2 diabetes was doing what it had to do - progressively rise. Endocrinologists like Gerry Reaven at Stanford University could see it happening. They even had a name for it - Syndrome X - but their voices could barely be heard over the roar of the low-cholesterol/reduced-fat avalanche.

And in the midst of all this "low cholesterol hoopla," drugs designed for the purpose of lowering cholesterol were to become the darlings of the pharmaceutical industry. Potentially millions, then billions, of dollars of profit were to be made from statin drugs.

These same drug company researchers soon devised more and more effective statin drugs. In time, the truly effective ones--Baycol®, Lipitor®, Lescol®, Pravachol®, Mevacor®, and Zocor®--were developed, some capable of as much as a 40 percent reduction of LDL cholesterol in just a matter of weeks. More recently, Vytorin® (just Zocor in disguise) and Crestor® have been introduced with an even greater claim for potency. So it has been only quite recently that these serious, even lethal, statin side effects have begun to emerge in a public and medical community lulled into complacency by ultra-positive direct-to-patient advertising and inexcusable misinformation.

The FDA prudently but somewhat belatedly "rushed" Baycol® off the market after two years because of dozens of rhabdomyolysis deaths. Rhabdomyolysis deaths are still occurring, albeit at a much-reduced rate. Even so, the numbers of rhabdomyolysis deaths from Lipitor®, Zocor® and

Mevacor®, Pravachol® and Crestor® now far exceed those from Baycol® alone. All of this for the purpose of lowering the blood level of the substance, cholesterol, that was already known to be absolutely vital for the human body to function. Even our very thought processes demand adequate supplies of this ubiquitous substance. And all of this pharmaceutical legerdemain is being done to control this wonder substance - which only occasionally winds up in atheroma because of misdirected "oxidized" lipoprotein - and which has no demonstrable causative role in arteriosclerosis.

And now we find that such health care dignitaries as John Abramson MD of Harvard, Jerome Hoffman of UCLA and David Brown MD of Albert Einstein and Beth Israel, in a letter to NIH dated 23 Sep 2004, charged complete lack of objectivity of the originators of the latest NCEP guidelines due to financial ties with the drug industry and criticized these guidelines for gross lack of scientific validation. George Mann MD of the Framington Study has previously called this misguided pre-occupation with cholesterol causality "a cholesterol scam" and the "greatest scientific deception of our times" [12].

Cholesterol is not the enemy, inflammation is and our statin drugs, despite their benefit as inhibitors of inflammation, were designed originally to interfere with the mevalonate pathway and therein lay the problem. In inhibiting the mevalonate pathway of cholesterol synthesis, statins inevitably must inhibit our glial cell cholesterol,

CoQ10 and ubiquinone, all so vital to the function of our bodies and minds – a terrible price to pay for inhibition of a substance now generally accepted to have no significant role in cardiovascular disease. Think about it!

CHAPTER 9
A Failed National Diet. What Diet Then?

If the low fat, low cholesterol, all too liberal refined carbohydrate diet of the past 40 years has failed, leaving statin drug use and vascular surgery of one type or another at an all time high, where do we turn? What do we do? Our past leaders seem to have failed us. Who, then, is qualified to take the lead?

Dr. Kilmer McCully's far-reaching conclusion - that natural cholesterol is innocuous to arteries and elevated homocysteine, not cholesterol, is one of the major causes of arteriosclerosis - naturally led him to re-examine every facet of the prevailing public food habits. In regard to the FDA's diet guidelines, he unequivocally states:

"The Food Pyramid is wrong on two counts: First, it is based on the false premise that cholesterol and saturated fats are the underlying cause of coronary heart disease. Second, it erroneously implies that all carbohydrates - whether refined or from whole food - are preferable to fats[1]."

One has but to look on the bookshelves of the local library and nutrition stores to observe that McCully is hardly alone in his philosophy. There are now many readable and informative books dealing with the subject of how our past decades of diet and nutrition standards have failed us. They very capably present the novel carbohydrate restrictive diet that McCully knew had to replace the old, national diet of the past. The first of these renegade leaders to gain notoriety is Dr. Robert C. Atkins but he was hardly the first to observe the problems inherent in the excessive reliance on carbohydrates in one's diet.

In 1892, the famous Dr. William Harvey imposed the then radical carbohydrate restrictive diet on his obese patient and friend, William Banting, with outstanding success. Banting lost over 40 pounds and, delighted, he wrote and published at his own expense his now famous Letter of Corpulence. Banting maintained a normal weight on his low carbohydrate diet[2] until his death at 81.

Atkins, a young cardiologist in 1963, found that for him a low carbohydrate diet worked to assuage his hunger and control his tendency to gain weight. He went on to write his famous book, now in its third edition, on the protein augmented, carbohydrate restrictive diet[3].

Atkins has been followed by legions of other writers rebelling against the guidelines and even the dictates of organized medicine represented by the United States Department of Agriculture (USDA), the American Diabetes Association (AbdA), the U.S. Food and Drug Administration (FDA), the National Cholesterol Education Program (NCEP), the National Heart, Lung and Blood Institute (NHLBI), and the Canadian Food Inspection Agency (CFIA). The millions of book sales these various authors have racked up against such odds reflect the awareness of the general public that all is not well with our food industry and national nutrition policies.

Joel Kauffman recently reviewed 12 of these popular books, comparing their strengths and weaknesses[4]. Kauffman describes the two books of this group which do not contain menus or recipes, one by Braly and Hoggan[5], and one by Ottoboni and Ottoboni[6] as both excellent and complementary. He describes the homocysteine and oxycholesterol portions of the McCully and McCully [7] book as excellent and complementary to the foregoing ones. He praises a book by Berstein[8] as being in a class by itself and must reading for diagnosed diabetics. For people not sure of which diet-based affliction they have, Kauffman encourages a book by Smith[9].

For overweight people who want minimal reading and a simple diet plan to follow, the Allan and Lutz[10] or Grove[11] books are recommended. The Eades and Eades[12] and Atkins[13] books are for those seeking more information and diet plans. Kauffman even considers the special dietary concerns of those from eastern Europe when he guides readers to a book by Kwasniewski and Chylinski[14].

In light of present knowledge, any one of these diets, if reasonably followed, will result in a general level of nutrition far superior to any served up by the low cholesterol, low fat doctrine during our past 50 years of homage.

And the slowly turning tide back to the natural fats that were the foundation of the American diet before the "prudent diet" became the national one is discussed in a paper by Mary Enig and Sally Fallon[15]. In "The Oiling of America" the authors offer a provocative and illuminating explanation of why the natural fats of our past diet - the butter, whole milk, lard and tallow - have been almost completely replaced in our society by the unnatural, highly processed vegetable oils loaded with the trans fats that are now competing with cholesterol as public health enemy No. 1.

Of particular interest is Enig and Fallon's account of the famous heart surgeon, Dr. Dudley White, and his stance on the diet controversy. The "prudent diet" proponents of the low fat/cholesterol juggernaut crushed his 1956 nationally televised plea for nutritional common sense into oblivion. Dr. White noted that heart disease in the form of myocardial infarction (MI) was non-existent in 1900 when egg consumption was high and corn oil was unavailable. When pressed to support the prudent diet, he replied, "See here, I began my practice as a cardiologist in 1921 and never saw a myocardial infarction patient until 1928. Back in the MI-free days before 1920, the fats were butter and lard, and I think we would all benefit from the kind of diet that we had at a time when no one had ever heard of corn oil." Today most people have forgotten all about Dr. Dudley White and his prophetic words of advice but we are now in a dietary revolution, and the natural fats of our grandparents are rightfully back in vogue in most of the cholesterol restrictive diets reviewed by Kauffman.

However, the Heart Revolution Diet outlined in Dr. McCully's book, *The Heart Revolution*[16], reflecting, as it does, his vast clinical research and conclusions, prompted us to focus on his dietary recommendations for the purpose of this book.

Dr. McCully's persistent, even tenacious, adherence to his almost "Eureka" concept of homocysteine toxicity causation of arteriosclerosis has gained wide acceptance from researchers in the field. From his first lonely review of arteriosclerotic changes in children who died from genetically pre-ordained homocystinuria, he now seems to have proven his point: cholesterol is not the cause of arteriosclerosis, inflammation is and homocysteine elevation secondary to vitamin deficiency appears to be a major player. Needless to say, to depart so radically from prevailing concepts takes a man with determination but it does not stop there.

McCully's historic work also points to vitamin deficiencies as playing the primary contributory role in arteriosclerosis. Homocysteine, the new villain, becomes predictably elevated in the body only when one or more of the B complex vitamins - folic acid, B6 or B12 - are deficient. The arteriosclerosis of homocysteine elevation, it would seem, is a deficiency disease, which, according to McCully (and now many others) makes it potentially treatable by dietary supplementation. Cholesterol is not completely off the hook but its role, when sufficiently elevated, has now become one of passive incorporation into atherosclerotic plaque. Most authorities now accept these findings but are quick to point out homocysteine elevation, by itself, cannot account for all arteriosclerosis and atherosclerosis observed.

As presented by Fallon and Enig in their paper on heart disease causation[17] and Kauffman in his review on supplements[18], other factors such as trans fats, unnatural omega-3/omega-6 ratios, insufficient magnesium, anti-oxidant deficiency, platelet malfunction, and even low levels of coenzyme Q10 may be involved. Certainly the concept of vitamin or mineral deficiencies as a cause or a significant contributor to public ill health is not new, but this major departure from traditional thinking, thanks in part to Dr. McCully untiring efforts, now has widespread research support.

Now, another deficiency state with major repercussions must be added to our already long list of serious diseases now proven to come from a nutritional deficiency origin. Our big killer – arteriosclerosis and its offspring, atherosclerosis, results from subtle deficiencies of such substances as folic acid, B6 and B12, the lack of which leads to toxic elevation of homocysteine levels.

McCully makes his case well, for these common substances - so vital for our ability to metabolize homocysteine - are not only exquisitely sensitive to our techniques of food preparation and processing but often become progressively less available to our bodies as we age. It can be stated unequivocally that despite the abundance of food in our burgeoning supermarkets, we are a nation in which many individuals are largely compromised by subtle deficiencies of folic acid, B6 and B12. The result is rampant arterial disease with its heart attacks and strokes, our most common cause of death and disability. It seems ironic that a country so favored with such a rich array of resources can suffer diseases caused by something so prosaic as completely preventable vitamin deficiencies. Any doctor worth his salt in public health administration and delivery of health care cringes at the thought.

The FDA's inaction on the vitamin supplementation issues was another factor in our recommendation of McCully's Heart Revolution Diet. In his discussion of the carbohydrate restrictive diet, McCully devotes special attention to foods that have abundant amounts of folic acid and the B6 and B12 vitamins so important for holding homocysteine in check. He also advises the necessary cooking techniques that minimize the loss of these substances during food preparation. He generally goes along with the mid-section of the Food Pyramid but recommends a few modifications. Although milk, cheese and yogurt are good sources of calcium and protein and the recommendation to eat two or three servings per day is valid, he takes issue with the recommendation to eat only low fat or fat free products. He is concerned about the associated risk of deficiency of fat-soluble vitamins, since these nutrients are found only in the fat portion of the foods we eat.

Another area McCully would modify is the FDA recommendation to consume two or three servings of meat, poultry, fish, dry beans, eggs or nuts a day. Putting beans and nuts in this group is problematic, he says, because it suggests that plant and animal proteins are interchangeable: "The truth is that plant protein, lacking in the essential amino acids, is quite different from animal protein, which contains plentiful essential amino acids. Therefore, depending only on plants for protein is not a good idea because the protein is inferior." He suggests a daily intake of two or three servings of protein from fish, meats, poultry, eggs or cheese.

He agrees with eating more vegetables and fruits, which are an excellent source of vitamins, minerals, fiber and complex carbohydrates, but reminds us that although "carbohydrates are essential we must choose beneficial carbohydrates-- fruits, vegetables and whole grains--not refined carbohydrates like sugar and flour products." He deplores the tendency of so many Americans to turn to highly refined, vitamin and mineral depleted, readily available, processed foods, which, for the most part, tend to be high in refined carbohydrates. As stated earlier, that excessive reliance on such carbohydrates in our diet has lead to the present carbohydrate catastrophe, the obesity epidemic.

McCully's diet is simple: Protein in the form of meat, fish, poultry, eggs, milk, cheese and beans should comprise about 25 percent of our daily caloric intake. Another 25 to 30 percent should come from the consumption of fats, which includes the fat of ingested meats plus olive oil, butter and cream. The remaining 45-50 percent of our daily caloric intake should be derived from the consumption of complex carbohydrates in the form of fruit, vegetables and whole grains. Balance is key in this diet, primary to maintaining balance in the body.

You won't find Oreos or white bread or French-fries in McCully's diet but you will find some remarkable similarities to the food nutritionists who postulate what our diet must have been like 10,000 years ago. Not only has McCully focused his diet on the prevention of arteriosclerosis but he also presents a diet to which we are already well suited, genetically speaking. We are still hunter-gathers like our forebears, he says, but we must now confine our searches to the aisles of supermarkets in our quest for just the right foods.

Not only does McCully's diet help keep homocysteine levels comfortably in the normal range, lessening the possibility of damage to the lining of our arteries, it also seems to be just as effective as the low cholesterol/low fat diet for normalizing serum cholesterol, a subject of immense concern to today's patients, despite the lack of any significant association with cardiovascular disease. If one's arteries are not primed with lipid streaks and foam cells, LDL remains in its largely unoxidized form, and cholesterol deposition into incipient atheroma becomes unlikely.

The overwhelming majority of people in our country today have been taught to regard cholesterol as the villain in coronary heart disease. Understandably, they have been led to consider the American Heart Association's low cholesterol/ low fat diet as the correct choice for keeping cholesterol levels in check. Because of this, they have become fair game for the promoters of broader and broader utilization of the statin class of drugs to reduce cholesterol levels. The reality that almost all major intervention studies have failed to find a significant correlation of serum cholesterol levels with cardiovascular diseases has fallen on ears deafened by drug promotional literature. Most individuals with the risk factors of hypertension, obesity, smoking and positive family history for arteriosclerosis now consider themselves to be suitable candidates for statin drug intervention despite their frequently modest cholesterol and LDL levels. This makes the job of those promoting wider use of statin drugs even easier.

Now we have learned that cholesterol is not the villain in arteriosclerosis - other factors are, primary of which is inflammation, secondary to homocysteine elevation among other causes. Our extraordinary efforts over the past fifty years to adhere to a low fat/ low cholesterol diet appear to have been misdirected. This recent evidence suggests, even demands, a radical departure from our dependence on a misguided "national" diet that not only has failed to nourish and protect our health but also has actively undermined it. We need a new diet that is far more restrictive with respect to the consumption of simple carbohydrates and processed foodstuffs that have been stripped of vitally important vitamins and minerals. Authorities are surely beginning to realize that, had we taken this path fifty years ago, our current dependence on statin drugs for control of heart disease and stroke would be substantially reduced, if not eliminated.

It is for this reason that I felt compelled to include social emphasis on diet in my presentation of the diverse side effects of the statin class of drugs. McCully has given us reason to believe that, while cholesterol is an absolutely vital substance, it is innocuous in its natural, unoxidized form. Its passive involvement as a component in sclerotic plaques occurs only because of pre-existing factors completely unrelated to cholesterol. If we are to rationally approach the problems of prevention of arteriosclerosis and its secondary complications of heart disease and stroke and excessive dependence on statin drugs, we need to recognize the full array of nutritional factors and inflammatory factors that are contributing. To accomplish this, anti-inflammatory supplements and proper diet must go hand in hand. Together, they can become a very effective "double whammy" in the prevention and treatment of arteriosclerosis and its complications.

Applying these concepts one can look toward a future with a greatly reduced need for statin drug use. Do we really have a choice?

CHAPTER 10
Statin Alternatives

One thing I have learned over the past six years of research on this subject is that neither patient nor doctor fully understands the true scope of statin drug side effects. Therefore it is reasonable to review them before delving into any discussion of alternative treatment. If one's current treatment plan seems to be working with no significant problems, I can see little merit in changing. But how can an individual, even a doctor, make a truly enlightened decision unless the full range of possible statin effects are known. Many people might fail to see a relationship between tingling in their fingers, depression, amyotrophic lateral sclerosis or hostility and their statin medication. Even their doctors may not have been adequately informed about many of the more subtle effects that have been reported. The following few paragraphs should help.

Transient global amnesia, forgetfulness, confusion, disorientation and increase of pre-existing senility represent only inhibition of vital brain cell cholesterol by the statin class of drugs. Cholesterol is also the precursor for synthesis of our sex hormones resulting in impaired sexuality, both erectile dysfunction and loss of libido, and reports of this among statin users are common. Rarely will a patient bring up these kinds of problems spontaneously.

What about the inevitable collateral damage to ubiquinones (CoQ10) and dolichols from use of these drugs? Any drug that inhibits the production of cholesterol via the mevalonate pathway, as all statins do, must also inhibit ubiquinones and dolichols.

Those from Co-Q10 inhibition give rise to liver inflammation, muscle inflammation known as myopathy with muscle ache, pain, sensitivity and soreness anywhere in the body and myopathy's more serious form, rhabdomyopathy with actual breakdown of muscle cells and secondary kidney blockage. When myopathy strikes the chest wall muscles, hundreds of patients have received expensive and worrisome cardiac workups.

Another complex of symptoms from CoQ10 inhibition results from neuropathy with ringing in the ears, vertigo, weakness of extremities, numbness, decreased ability to feel heat or cold and altered sensation anywhere in the body – numbness and tingling of the feet being a common early sign. Such symptoms are common in our elderly and their special association with statin drug use is easily missed.

Lack of sufficient CoQ10 dependant energy reserves results in tiredness, shortness of breath and easy fatigability and congestive heart failure with ankle edema, nocturia, shortness of breath with recumbency and the need for extra pillows for sleep. Seniors are especially prone to have such symptoms and be unaware of a possible relationship to their statin drug.

These are only some of the more common side effects of CoQ10 deficiency. Physicians for the most part are well aware of hepatitis, myopathy and rhabdomyolysis but many still steadfastly refuse to admit neuropathy despite the convincing published works of David Gaist of the University of Southern Denmark in Odense. And cardiologists and internists still deny the reality of congestive heart failure from excessive CoQ10 inhibition despite the widely published and equally convincing research of the Doctors Peter and Alena Langsjoen of Texas. These dedicated cardiologists have been researching this subject for years.

Additional symptoms we now associate with statin induced dolicol inhibition, include a broad range of affective disorders, reflecting alteration of neuropeptides, known as brain cell messengers. Dolichols are absolutely necessary for the formation of these neuropeptides, known also as messenger molecules. These short chains of peptides not only are the basis of every thought, emotion and sensation we have ever experienced; they are our every thought, emotion or sensation in a process we are only just beginning to understand.

"He or she is not the person I married," is a frequently recurring statement from spouses of statin users. And more ominously is the statement from surviving wives, "There was nothing wrong before his statin. I know that drug killed him."

Very few physicians and almost no patients are aware of the many case reports of statin associated hostility, aggression, combativeness, homicidal feelings, road-rage type behavior, accident and addiction proneness and depression of varying degrees with its inevitable suicidal ideation, attempts and occasional successes.

The relationship of such symptoms with statin drug use is all too frequently missed and written off as "emotional" and therefore nothing to do with their statin. Yet there is another even more obscure group of diagnoses associated with statin drug use, the development of certain neurodegenerative diseases. Parkinson's disease, amyotrophic lateral sclerosis (ALS) frontal lobe dementia and multiple system abnormalities are being reported with unusual frequency among statin users and researchers have found a likely explanation – abnormal tau protein, another area of collateral damage from mevalonate pathway interference. Please refer to the Addendum section for more on this important subject.

So when a physician asks someone if they are having any problems with their statins, he must be specific, for when they have no awareness of what statins can do, patients are very unlikely to report such problems as depression and hostility, even if severe. As to their memory impairment, Muldoon tells us that much cognitive loss passes unnoticed, even by the statin impaired victim. Something to think about, isn't it?

a. Coenzyme Q-10 Supplementation

The importance of mitochondrial function in meeting the energy needs of the heart has been emphasized recently because of the increasing tendency towards congestive heart failure (CHF) in statin drug users. Cardiologist Dr. Peter Langsjoen, MD, has published a number of articles on this subject and reviewed the prevalence of statin-associated CHF in many controlled studies, reporting on the prompt response of CHF to supplemental CoQ10 or substantial reductions in statin dosage[1,2]. Statin drugs, as HMG-CoA reductase inhibitors of the critical mevalonate pathway, must inevitably curtail the availability of CoQ10, vital to mitochondrial function, energy production and the very structure of every cell in our body[3]. The heart is often the first to feel the effects of lack of energy because of its extraordinary energy demands as a pump but every cell in our bodies is just as dependent upon ubiquinone-fueled mitochondria.

Like man's evolution of the gasoline engine to power billions of complicated mechanical devices including the ubiquitous automobile, nature has evolved the ATP mechanism for powering most, if not all, of life's myriad of energy requirements. This entire ATP generating process is ultimately dependant upon abundant reserves of ubiquinone; the same offspring of the mevalonate pathway critically curtailed by statin drugs.

In the June 2004 issue of Archives of

Neurology, the Neurology Department of Columbia University reported a greater than 50% fall in plasma coenzyme Q10 in their group taking Lipitor 80 mg for 30 days - a striking documentation of the impact of statin therapy on CoQ10 biosynthesis. Others studies have shown that even more modest doses of our powerful statins progressively erode our CoQ10 availability. This inevitable collateral damage is a major contributor to intolerable, dangerous and even lethal statin side effects.

In addition to its critically important role in energy production, CoQ10 has a possibly even greater role within the mitochondria as an anti-oxidant[4,5], with a free radical-quenching ability some 50 times greater than that of vitamin E.

Yet the most fundamental role of CoQ10 is in the structure of our cell walls. Body cells can function properly only the walls of each cell have sufficient tension and stability. Insufficiency of CoQ10 results in the cell wall breakdown we commonly see as statin associated hepatitis and myopathy and may possibly contribute to statin associated neuropathy and neurodegenerative diseases as well.

The adult human body pool of this substance has been reported to be 2 grams, and requires replacement of about 0.5 gram per day[6,7]. This must be supplied by endogenous synthesis or dietary intake. Synthesis decreases progressively in humans as we grow older and the average CoQ10 content of the western diet is less than 5 mg/day. Thus, CoQ10 supplementation appears to be the only way for older people to obtain their daily need of this important nutrient. Nearly 40 million people will be taking Lipitor this year in the United States alone, with an additional 20 million taking other types of statin drugs of comparable effect. Most of these people will be over 50 years of age, but few of them will be on supplemental CoQ10. Simple logic dictates that the statin drug impact on ubiquinone availability and mitochondrial energy production will be profound.

Dosage of CoQ10 depends on the condition. If you are using it with your statin merely to prevent the onset of muscles aches and pains or nerve damage, a dose of 100 to 200mg daily is reasonable. On the other hand, if you already have these problems and have stopped your statin drug and are trying to get back to normal, a daily dose of 500mg or more might be advisable, especially since Q10 is a very safe, natural substance. It is true also that in selected clinical trials of certain neurological conditions, such as Parkinson's disease, doses up to 2400mg daily are being studied with little to no evidence of side effects. As to the best form of this important supplement, try to find Gelcaps and look for economy.

b. Omega 3 and Inflammation

On the subject of what we can do for arterial inflammation, Lee of the Thrombosis and Vascular Biology Unit of Birmingham's City Hospital in the U.K., strongly recommends omega-3 in the long-term treatment plan of his myocardial infarction patients and brilliantly presents his documentation[1]. There is no longer any doubt as to the vital role of this polyunsaturated fatty acid in reducing cardiovascular disease risk. Not only has it been firmly documented to stabilize the myocardium electrically, resulting in reduced ventricular arrhythmias and sudden death but also it has been found to have potent anti-inflammatory effects quite comparable to those of the statin drugs.

Our omega 3's are fatty acids that our body derives from food. Studies have discovered that omega-3 fatty acids have anti-inflammatory effect due to their ability to convert into anti-inflammatory prostaglandins[2,3]. In addition, omega-3 fatty acids can decrease the production of inflammatory prostaglandins by omega 6, resulting in a greater decrease in inflammation.

Omega-3s are essential fatty acids, vital for human health. There are two families of essential fatty acids: omega-3 fatty acids and omega-6 fatty acids. They are termed "essential" because they cannot be produced by the body, and must therefore be obtained from the diet.

Our typical Western diet has evolved to be high in omega-6 and relatively low in omega-3 fatty acids. While omega-6 fatty acids are not necessarily bad, a skewed ratio in favor of too much omega-6 can be detrimental to one's health by allowing the production of excess inflammatory prostaglandins. A balance of omega-6 and omega-3 fatty acids is essential for proper health. Research is still underway to define the precise mechanism by which omega 3 exerts its beneficial effect on reduction of cardiovascular disease risk. Our most important established truth is that the ratio of omega 3 to omega 6 in our diet has been falling for decades, closely paralleling the rise in heart disease during the same time period.

The recommended dose of omega-3 is quite variable, for there is no established upper limit to this vital yet essentially harmless food substance.
My recommendation is for at least 1200 mg of omega-3 supplementation daily as a routine, in the form of fish in your diet, fish oil capsules or its equivalent from other sources of omega-3. If on the basis of family or personal history, one is high risk for cardiovascular disease, at least doubling this amount should be considered.

c. The Role of the B Vitamins

Not only did McCully focus on the observation that homocysteinuria in children created a condition seemingly identical to the arteriosclerosis of the elderly[1] but he also knew of the work of George Spaeth, an ophthalmologist friend, who informed him of the dramatically beneficial effect of vitamin B6 supplementation on some of the homocysteinuria patients he had treated. Spaeth reported to McCully his observation that the excretion of homocysteine in the urine of such patients frequently could be increased dramatically by vitamin B6. Two seeds were thereby planted in Kilmer McCully's receptive mind: the amino acid homocysteine, if elevated, causes a condition remarkably like arteriosclerosis; and a simple vitamin, B6, could lower homocysteine levels.

Some time later at another genetics conference, McCully learned of another homocystinuria-like case: a two-month-old baby that had died despite aggressive attempts at therapy. This time, the urine contained both homocysteine and another substance called cystathionine, also related to homocysteine. In the case of this unfortunate baby, its metabolic passageway was deficient in a different enzyme and the conversion would have required vitamin B12. When McCully examined the slides of the baby's arteries he found the same arteriosclerosis changes noted in all the previous cases.

McCully went on to discover that folic acid also shared this homocysteine protective role and was yet another vitamin, which, if deficient, could cause one's homocysteine to rise. He then went on to study the levels of these critical vitamins in various population groups and soon defined substantial numbers of people genetically deficient in one or more of the vitamins due to enzymatic mutations. In other mostly older groups, he found acquired deficiencies of B6, 12 or folic acid. Soon he had demonstrated that in our population at large, deficiencies of one or more of these three vitamins were remarkably common. His ground-breaking work soon was corroborated by others[2,3,4].

Kilmer McCully recommends the following daily doses of these readily available and economic B vitamins for reasonable homocysteine control:
Vitamin B6 – 80-100mg
Vitamin B12 – 200-250mcg
Folic Acid – 400-800mcg

d. Why a Buffered Baby Aspirin?

You would think by now the aspirin issue had long ago been put to rest. Yet the debate still continues with the primary care physician right in the center, trying to decide which tune to follow.

Three decades ago, right in the middle of my 23 year "tour of duty" as a family doctor, the general consensus, the tune to which we all danced, was that for all males over the age of 50 (and probably women as well), the benefits of a baby aspirin daily far outweighed possible risks.

It seemed logical that inhibition of platelets, the proven mechanism of action of aspirin in men would be helpful in both primary and secondary prevention of myocardial infarctions and although women may come from Venus and men from Mars, I never saw any strong reason to withhold this medication from women.

The problem here again is that fellow named Gauss and his frequency distribution curve. You give 81 mg of aspirin (baby aspirin dose) to a thousand people and 25 of them will likely bleed excessively into their tissues and return to the office looking like victims of physical assault, another 25 will have no effect on platelets whatsoever, demonstrating complete insensitivity to aspirin at that dose and the rest will be in the middle, some leaning right and some left.

That is what makes medicine an art rather than a science. Our DNA mandate is such that no two of us are alike and that goes for reactions to medicines of all kinds. So in public health as in primary and secondary prevention, you try to find the middle road when there is no such thing.

And now we find that the results of longitudinal studies of large numbers of people are not nearly as supportive of aspirin as we once thought. I have heard doctors say as they go off for their year of self-sacrifice into third world countries, "You give me all the salt, penicillin and aspirin I need and I can practice medicine anywhere." They have now taken away penicillin with threats of dire sensitivity reactions and limited spectrum of effectiveness. What if they take away our aspirin? How much can you do with salt? – quite a lot actually but that is another story.

Now, thanks to Joel Kauffman's critical review[1], we find that much has changed. First of all, the buffer coating on aspirin has proven to be critical for its vital magnesium content. Secondly, after critical appraisal of side effects and all cause death rates, the use of low dose aspirin in primary prevention can no longer be supported.

Secondary prevention is quite another matter with very favorable outcomes for limited periods of times after the thrombotic event. The trouble is, one never knows when a person evolves from primary to secondary for the transition may be completely silent – a bit of subendothelial inflammation. Until a thrombotic event occurs there is no announcement that this individual's status has now changed from primary (aspirin no) to secondary (aspirin yes).

Thankfully, this still fits with our knowledge of relevant pathophysiology - the inhibition of platelet stickiness by aspirin. In secondary prevention you are dealing with an endothelial wound and aspirin during the healing period seems reasonable.

In primary prevention there is no wound – this is a different kind of problem. So our challenge for rational aspirin use seems to be one of identifying those patients at risk, those with open endothelial lesions or those very likely to have them. From the viewpoint of a family doctor charged with responsibility for his patient's health and since reliable markers of inflammation are not as yet available, many primary care physicians will opt for aspirin's use in primary prevention regardless, especially since a single baby aspirin has so few side effects

Since we now better understand the vital role of inflammation in atherosclerosis we are in need of better markers of inflammation to guide our identification of those at risk. Our CRP is a step in that direction but a much better marker is necessary. With such a marker we physicians would have little doubt in determining which patients to place on aspirin and the "super-aspirins" to follow now that we are focusing on the true etiology of atherosclerosis.

On this subject of inflammation, we are indebted to Kauffman's suggestion of such aspirin substitutes as omega 3, Co-enzyme Q10, magnesium and even vitamin E, all of which address inflammation at least as effectively as aspirin, if not more so, and do so with near absence of side effects.

The benefits of vitamin E and magnesium are referenced by Kauffman in his review of aspirin compared with other modalities for both primary and secondary prevention of cardiovascular disease. Kauffman cites the special effectiveness of Bufferin because of the magnesium content of the enteric coating, which supplements the established benefit of low-dose aspirin.

e. Low Dose Statins

Now that the results of long-term studies of statin use have been published, few would argue statin drug's effectiveness in reducing cardiovascular disease risk. To be sure, other substances having nothing or little to do with our alleged nemesis, cholesterol, also have demonstrated considerable benefit in this regard. Such therapies include omega 3, Coenzyme-Q10, vitamins B6, B12 and folic acid, anti-oxidants and even buffered aspirin.

But in considering only the statins, study after study has shown the benefit of these agents in reducing the risk of heart attack and stroke, especially when used for secondary prevention. However, almost buried in this barrage of positive results is our growing research evidence that this reduction of cardiovascular disease morbidity and mortality from statin use has occurred independently of cholesterol effect.

Regardless of the cholesterol level of the subject at the start of statin therapy, whether normal or high and regardless of the level of cholesterol reduction, whether great or small or none at all, statins, originally felt to work solely as an inhibitor of cholesterol biosynthesis, appear to work independently of cholesterol.

Just what is going on here? Weren't we all taught years ago that only by decreasing serum cholesterol by haranguing our patients these past 35 years as to the merits of a low fat/low cholesterol diet and by writing expensive prescriptions for a long list of increasingly potent cholesterol "busting" drugs could we expect to reduce cardiovascular disease risk? And now we find statin benefit independently of any cholesterol factor. Isn't cholesterol still "public health enemy number one"? Can't we still use the "C" word to frighten small children?

Adding to this evolving puzzle about the cause of cardiovascular disease is the work of Kilmer McCully, who, despite massive obstacles of opposition to any concepts of arteriosclerosis and atherosclerosis contrary to a cholesterol causation, successfully demonstrated to the then reluctant scientific world that homocysteine elevation is a major player in cardiovascular disease, relegating cholesterol's appearance in plaques to that of an "innocent bystander". Adding to cholesterol's innocence is its vital role in our body - mediator of synaptic transmissions, precursor of vital hormones and the most abundant biochemical in our brains. Only in its unnatural, oxidized form does cholesterol exhibit toxicity.

Does this mean back to eggs and whole milk? Think about it!

The cholesterol of fresh eggs - harmless. That of powdered eggs - toxic! Cholesterol of whole milk - harmless. That of dried milk, so popular in the world - toxic! Sort of ruins your weekly shopping trip through the pastry aisles, doesn't it? Can you find even a cracker, free of the "oxy" form of cholesterol? I doubt it for most commercial chefs use powdered milk and eggs rather than the natural form!

Despite this evidence of a new non-cholesterol factor in cardiovascular disease risk, our nutritional and pharmaceutical world remains steadfastly focused on cholesterol, the villain. Most of our primary care physicians today, marching lockstep to drug company guidelines, prescribe whatever dose of powerful statins is required to lower serum cholesterol, even though this same cholesterol is increasingly considered to be irrelevant.

Statins work by another mechanism, drug company researchers now say. They relieve inflammation in the endothelial lining of blood vessels. And recently, the greedy eye of our statin "monster" (for that is what it has become in terms of economic and social impact) is focusing on extending the use of statins to organ transplant recipients and victims of autoimmune diseases. Why? Because they work!

To read Shovman's excellent review in Cutting Edge Reports[1] of "The anti-inflammatory and immuno-modulatory properties of statins", is like entering the topsy-turvy world of Alice in Wonderland, where the effect of lowering one's immune defenses, which most of us intuitively feel is of doubtful benefit, can be interpreted as good for the organ transplant recipient and autoimmune disease victim but bad for most infectious disease and cancer risk. One must admire this "positive spin" ability usually seen only in the Washington political arena.

The good I see from the large numbers of excellent studies having to do with this new statin role of attenuating our immune system is that the attention of our clinicians is now beginning to be focused on the true cause of arteriosclerosis and atherosclerosis and the realization will soon dawn that cholesterol is conspicuously absent in the "usual suspect" line-up.

When, we might ask, will the doctors who write the prescriptions begin to question the merit of a cholesterol-lowering dose of statin drug when cholesterol is not an issue? Although the results of the ongoing low dose statin trials will not be known for several years, we already have some tantalizing clues. One of the more relevant comes from Japan where Matsuzaki[2] reported the results of a 6-year follow up of 47,294 Japanese patients treated with low dose Zocor (5-10 mg daily) for their hypercholesterolemia. Most would consider statin doses in this range to be bordering on sub-therapeutic, yet even with this low statin dose, substantial lowering of cardiovascular disease mortality resulted. I cite this study as one of the very first to examine the effectiveness of low doses of statins on cardiovascular disease risk independently of cholesterol effect.

The paper by Hilgendorph A and others[3] reported in the International Journal of Clinical Pharmacology and Therapeutics in 2003, is a must read for anyone sincerely concerned with the relative anti-inflammatory effects of the various

110

statins in current use. Despite strident claims to the contrary, statements of relative strengths as they appear in drug literature rarely are "exactly true". In Hilgendorph's study, blood monocyte cells were incubated with 6 different statins. All statins demonstrated an inhibitory effect on NF-kappaB, with Baycol being the strongest inhibitor of NF-kappaB activity. Hilgendorph reported dosage dependent NK-kB inhibition with a relative potency order of: Baycol> Mevacor> Zocor> Lipitor> Pravachol> Lescol. Of special interest to me in perusing the various graphs and figures accompanying this article was their graph of dose vs. response for these various statins, showing a very substantial NF-kB inhibitory effect even at the lowest starting doses studied, with a logarithmic response rather than arithmetic. Statin doses higher than basal provoked less and less NF-kB inhibition, in a manner very similar to aspirin's inhibition of platelet activation, where 81mg is almost as effective as 325mg. Incidentally, this reaction also is mediated by NF-kB.

In 2003, Law and others[4] reported the remarkable effects of low dose statins on both LDL cholesterol and ischemic heart disease reduction in an impressive study reported in BMJ. One would have thought this comprehensive meta-analysis would have shaken the very foundation of the medical community with respect to dosing strategy of the statin drugs, yet all that was heard was an inaudible "ho-hum" as if nothing had registered. The authors of this impressive, to me, study reported that reductions in LDL cholesterol (in the 164 trials observed) were 2.8 mmol/l (60%) with rosuvastatin 80 mg/day, compared with 1.8 mmol/l (40%) with rosuvastatin 5 mg/day, all from pretreatment LDL cholesterol concentrations of 4.8 mmol/l. The cholesterol reductions from low dose therapy I consider irrelevant but what really impresses me is the risk reduction.

In the 58 trials where the effect of statins on ischemic heart disease was studied, Law reported that for an LDL cholesterol reduction of 1.0 mmol/l, the risk of IHD events was reduced by 11% in the first year of treatment, 24% in the second year, 33% in year three to five, and by 36% thereafter. Law predicted that after several years a reduction of 1.8 mmol/l of LDL cholesterol would reduce IHD events by an estimated 61%. His results from the same 58 trials, corroborated by results from the nine cohort studies, showed that lowering LDL cholesterol decreases all stroke by 10% for a 1 mmol/l reduction and 17% for a 1.8 mmol/l reduction.

Although the rest of the medical community may have "ho-hummed" Law's BMJ paper, the results astounded me. I am very impressed that rosuvastatin 5 mg daily, one sixteenth the size of the 80 mg dose, can give 61% of the ischemic heart disease reduction and 17% reduction in stroke risk. I can think of no stronger case for the consideration of low dose statins by our primay care physicians than this paper by Law. Obviously further studies are needed to define low dose response relationships but this is an excellent start.

Since the development of statin drugs, the end-point for judging effectiveness has been the cholesterol response. If cholesterol seemed reluctant to be lowered, a higher dosage of statin was the almost automatic response. Our focus on cholesterol as the culprit has led us to higher and higher statin dosages over the years as target levels for our serum cholesterol have been progressively lowered.

Today it is almost standard that the starting dose be at least 20 to 40 mg of Lipitor or Zocor, (or its equivalent in the other statins) and 80mg doses have become increasingly common. All of this we justified to further reduce our sometimes sluggish serum cholesterol in a research climate that almost daily reveals the increased irrelevancy of cholesterol.

Since cholesterol response no longer seems to be a valid end-point in determining statin dose, the entire strategy for dosing these drugs must be reviewed, using a marker of inflammation as endpoint, not cholesterol. The effectiveness of statins on cardiovascular disease risk at radically lower dosages must be defined.

Using Lipitor as an example, the relative benefit on cardiovascular disease of 5 mg and even 2.5 mg should be studied. As Jay Cohen has emphasized in his book, Over Dose, most side effects of the statin drugs would never have occurred if the philosophy, "start low, go slow" on statin dosing were applied.

The obvious problem with this philosophy is the apparent lack of a meaningful end-point that defines anti-inflammatory success. C-reactive protein is an inflammatory marker that has shown considerable usefulness in defining high risk for cardiovascular disease but unfortunately it is non-specific.

Inflammation anywhere in the body from chronic unsuspected infectious disease such as low-grade prostatitis, urethritis, cholecystis, gingivitis, cervicitis, or diverticulitis or even the onset of the common cold may trigger falsely positive CRP test results, meaningless in terms of underlying arterial inflammation.

A far more specific test when available for wide spread use may involve the increasingly well-known transcription factor, nuclear factor-kappa B (NF-kB). This vital substance appears to be the basis of our entire complex of anti-inflammatory and immuno-modulatory reactions. All statins have been proven to inhibit NF-kB, some far more strongly than others and it would seem that this reaction, or some corollary of it, if biochemically feasible, has a definite marker potential.

Although it is far too early to rejoice, there is compelling reason to believe that statin dosing considered miniscule by today's standards may yield effective anti-inflammatory activity with near absence of our present scourge of side effects.

f. Mother Nature's Statin

Red yeast rice is readily available in our country as a food supplement and as such it does not fall under FDA guidelines. The prevailing opinion about this substance is that since it is natural and uncontrolled it is generally safe to use. This is wrong. The first thing one must understand about red yeast rice is that it is just another statin.

One can imagine the chagrin of the pharmaceutical industry to discover in a simple yeast from the Orient, that Mother Nature already had provided her very own "completely natural" HMG- CoA inhibitor, red yeast rice! For thousands of years this yeast, known as Monascus purpureus, has been used to ferment rice into wine and as both a spice and preservative. Needless to say, any possible interference of this oriental fermentation product with our emerging statin drug industry was obviated by Merck's patent - the first ever filed on a naturally occurring substance. Mother Nature's cholestin would never compete with Merck's identical product, lovastatin, which has the trade name of Mevacor.

Red yeast rice[1] has been used in the Orient for hundred of years. Since 800 A.D. this substance has been employed by the Chinese as both a food and a medicine. Its therapeutic benefits as both a promoter of blood circulation and a digestive stimulant were first noted in the traditional Chinese pharmacopoeia, *Ben Cao Gang Mu-Dan Shi Bu Yi,* during the Ming Dynasty (1368–1644). In China, red yeast rice is used to treat abdominal pain due to what they call stagnant blood and dysentery, as well as for both external as well as internal trauma. In addition to its therapeutic applications, red yeast rice has been used for centuries as a flavor enhancer, a food preservative, and a base for a Taiwanese alcoholic rice-wine beverage.

The traditional method of making red yeast rice is to ferment the yeast naturally on a bed of cooked non-glutinous whole rice kernels. Recently this process has become industrialized. The active components of red yeast rice can vary considerably and the fermentation process demands strict vigilance to insure freedom from toxic impurities.

Red yeast rice contains numerous active constituents, including monacolin I to VI, monacolin K and dihydromonacolin, all of which have the same HMG-CoA reductase inhibitor effect as our modern statins. The only difference is that this product was made by Mother Nature long before our pharmaceutical industry conceived the idea and, allowing for some variations in composition from time to time, will reduce cardiovascular risk much like any of our pharmaceutical statins for it is lovastatin, Merck's generic name for its widely prescribed Mevacor.

When one takes red yeast rice they are effectively on statins and subject to all the purported benefits and side effects. I have had many cases of side effects from this "natural drug" reported to me. Myopathies and even our dreaded rhabdomyolysis have been reported from the use of Mother Nature's

116

red yeast rice. The issue is primarily one of dosage or, in some cases, co-administration of other drugs.

Since cholesterol response no longer seems to be a valid end-point in determining statin dose, the entire strategy for dosing all statins must be reviewed. The effectiveness of statins on cardiovascular disease risk at radically lower dosages must be defined. Since red yeast rice is just another statin, the same principles apply.

Red yeast rice is usually available in 400-600 mg size capsules with manufacturer's recommended beginning dose of 1-2 capsules twice daily. You will see occasional side effects at this dosage, especially with concurrent administration of erythromycin, grapefruit juice or especially if you are the recipient of tissue or organ transplant and are taking cyclosporin. This manufacturer's recommended dose is based upon cholesterol response, no longer considered a valid endpoint of statin effectiveness.

My strong recommendation to anyone considering the use of red yeast rice is that they take no more than one capsule daily combined with the other OTC anti-inflammatory supplements recommended in this chapter. Together with these other anti-inflammatory supplements, red yeast rice will give a powerful anti-inflammatory response. You will not see cholesterol reduction with this treatment plan nor should you be concerned, for inflammation, not cholesterol, is the true cause of increased cardiovascular risk. This treatment plan is of proven effectiveness for risk reduction with rare, if any, side effects.

CHAPTER 11
Conclusion

Transient global amnesia is probably as old as man and, as we have suggested, statin drugs may be just the latest of its many triggers. However, its varied reactions - vague preservation of identity, maddeningly repetitive questioning, absolute inability to preserve new memories and, in some cases, retrograde memory lapses decades into the past - can be subtle and elusive. But, as I have described in chapter 2 and in the following case report, regardless of which trigger provokes an attack - cold water, emotional stress, exercise, sex, cerebral angiography or statin drugs - the psychological impact on the patient is devastating!

"I was on four different statins for a period of over 10 years, on dosages from 10 mg to 80 mg. I had muscle pain and cramps for a number of years, and I put it down to aging or muscle strain. This was while I was on 10 mg to 40 mg. In July of 2002 I was on 40 mg of Pravachol®, and after blood tests showed [my] cholesterol was over 400, I was placed on 80 mg of Lipitor®. And that is when the nightmare began. Although the pain from muscle spasms and cramps had become so bad that I took early retirement in 2001 because I could not get through the day, I had never had problems with memory or cognitive functions before. I did not suspect statin drug toxicity until April 2003 when my husband suggested to my neurologist that I come off all meds for two weeks to see if that would help.

At that time the only way I could walk was with a cane or a walker to keep myself from falling. I had very little muscle tone in the calves of my legs, and my legs would just suddenly give way under me. And the pain was terrible.

Since going on the Lipitor® in July 2002, I have had four episodes of disoriented thinking, confusion and lost time. The last time occurred 6 August 2003 and lasted approximately 2 to 3 hours. The time before, I lost about 5 hours and that occurred on 22 June 2003. My husband and daughter took me to the ER that time.

I am so tired of defending myself from doctors who feel my problems do not have anything to do with the statins, and that everything that happened to me is "mental". I am at the point of not going back to see my primary care physician again or any other specialist. I definitely will not take their statins!"

This person has been devastated - emotionally, physically and mentally - by her experiences with statin drug use over the past 10 years. Clearly, she has experienced disabling physical symptoms but, in addition, she reports 4 amnesia episodes. She is an excellent example of the medical community's failure to recognize the full spectrum of statin drug side effects and to understand that many of them are irreversible.

Statin drugs, as they currently exist, interfere with cholesterol biosynthesis at the HMG-CoA reductase step and, as a consequence, inevitably must interfere with ubiquinone and dolichol production, processes vital for cell integrity, energy, anti-oxidation and neuropeptide synthesis. This can only be called collateral damage, a very serious consideration, since most of the side effects we are seeing are secondary to this collateral damage. Even the inhibition by statins of glial cell biosynthesis of brain cholesterol is collateral damage, unforeseen by the designers of statin drugs 20 years ago. Cognitive problems seem almost inevitable with interference of this vital glial cell role. Our dependence of neuronal transmission on glial cell synthesis of cholesterol was not known until Frank Pfrieger's landmark Science article of 2001. If our pharmaceutical industry was concerned by this astounding news from Pfrieger then you would never have known it. There is no evidence they even paused in their aggressive promotion of statins nor did they provide any special labeling on drug information pamphlets or encourage verbal warnings by drug "reps" to the thousands of unsuspecting physicians who are prescribing their statin drugs.

It is impossible to hide my frustration that now, long after patient case reports first began to surface, the average practicing physician in this country is still completely unaware that serious side effects can be associated with statin drug use. Many of those reports tell of doctors who, on hearing of memory gaps and increasing confusion, jump immediately to the presumptive diagnosis of "senior moments," approaching "senility" or possibly even "early Alzheimer's". Frequently, the last thing considered, if, indeed, the doctor thinks of it at all, is a reaction to the patient's statin drug. And the myriads of other complaints known to be associated with statin drug use - the depression, hostility, numbness and tingling, energy lack and sore muscles are much too often dismissed by the physician as "just a coincidence" or "to be expected at your age" and they just scoff at any possibility of Lou Gehrig's or Parkinson's disease .

My primary goal in writing this book will be realized when doctors first consider statin side effects as the genesis of these symptoms by their bewildered patients and reduce the dosage of the statin drug or stop the statin and seek an alternative therapy.

Doctors must also remember that such side effects do not necessarily become apparent only in the first few months of statin therapy. Some of the most serious side effects reported have presented after an interval of three or four trouble-free years of statin use, so constant vigilance is necessary.

Patients all too frequently accept erosion of memory and increasing tendency for confusion and disorientation as an inevitable consequence of aging. They, too, often need to be reminded that not all memory, emotional, muscle and nerve problems are age related and that they as well as their doctors must always consider a medication's side effects when these kinds of problems appear.

And there are two sides to the cholesterol issue. This notorious, Janus-faced substance is both a component of atherosclerotic plaque and, at the same time, one of the most important substances in our body. In its first guise, there is no doubt that cholesterol is found in atheroma but it is not the cause of the underlying arterial disease. McCulley[1] helped pave the way - and other researchers are following - when he determined that homocysteine, by allowing lipid/mucoid 'streaks' and inflammatory cells to accumulate in those fragile tissues lining the arteries, is an important initial trigger of atherosclerosis in many cases. Research results including those from our many longitudinal studies have now proven what McCully so persistently suspected – inflammation, not cholesterol, is the cause of atherosclerosis. Cholesterol is a more or less passive bystander, streaming by these damaged areas within its lipoprotein carrier and occasionally deposited by errant LDL, misguided in its alien, "oxidized" form. Gobbled up by a wandering phagocyte, the complex becomes the ominous "foam cell" and the process of hardening of the arteries with plaque formation is underway. With or without excess cholesterol the process of arteriosclerosis and atherosclerosis can and does take place in arteries. Homocysteine and other arterial toxins are the true triggers of this inflammatory process, not cholesterol.

Strong statins such as Lipitor®, Mevacor® Crestor®, Zocor® and its combined form, Vytorin®, have the capacity to cause major reductions in serum cholesterol values. Many patients proudly announce that their cholesterol plummeted "from 280 to 160" in a matter of weeks, attesting to the spectacular effectiveness of these stronger statins in some patients but we must remember that with the exception of Crestor® and Pravachol®, they tend to be lipophilic, easily traversing the so-called blood brain barrier, which for these statins is no barrier at all. And the hydrophilicity of Crestor® and Pravachol® is incomplete – cognitive side effects still occur. Dr. Beatrice Golomb, of UCSD's Department of Medicine, reports that in her case studies of transient global amnesia patients[3], cholesterol reductions of 100 points or more were very common. Such evidence suggests that abrupt, major decreases of serum cholesterol from statin drug therapy should be taken more as a warning than as an indication of success, for cognitive side effects seemed more likely to occur in these cases. When the practicing physician, who, despite the paucity of supportive research data, has determined that the use of statin drugs for cholesterol control is justified, is faced with this type of response, consideration should be given to prompt reduction in statin drug dosage of these patients, followed by more gradual titration to the lowest possible effective dose. Such patients are unusually sensitive to the statin class of drugs and special attention to dosage is required to minimize side effects. For many medications, one-half or one-quarter of the recommended starting dose may be completely adequate for patients, Dr. Jay Cohen[4] advises, and this lower amount will give comparable results with fewer side effects. The statin drugs, if used for cholesterol control, are no exception and the dosages are cumulative in their effect. The longer even the smaller doses are taken by a patient, however, the more potent they can become, and care must be exercised on an on-going basis to further reduce even maintenance doses if necessary.

As Cohen advises, "With all drugs, doctors should prescribe the smallest dose possible that will achieve the desirable goal of reasonable control." Defining reasonable control of serum cholesterol levels is not easy in light of the failure of study after study to show a significant effect on all cause mortality. An excellent review of this dilemma is presented by John Allred in his review article on lowering serum cholesterol.[5] In light of our present knowledge of cholesterol's largely passive role in arteriosclerosis and the very substantial side effect risks from the stronger statin drugs, attempts to reduce the risk of cardiovascular disease by cholesterol control may be counterproductive for many patients. This may be particularly true in patients who have no other serious medical issues.

We naturally focused our attention on diet, as the shift in scientific thinking toward homocysteine elevation as the cause of arteriosclerosis, and the importance of folic acid, B6 and B12 in controlling homocysteine levels in the body became evident. The "national" low cholesterol/low fat diet has failed not only its original intent to control arteriosclerosis and its consequences, it has actually fueled Type 2 diabetes and obesity epidemics in this country. In its race to produce low cholesterol and low fat products to satisfy that national diet, the food industry has delivered a superabundance of refined carbohydrates and nutrient-depleted foodstuffs that have exacerbated the problem. Instead of healthier, we have become a generation of pathetically "fattened sheep," prey to diabetes, stroke, heart attack, and worsening arteriosclerosis.

For these very real dietary reasons, we have stressed the importance of Dr. Kilmer McCully's research efforts over the past decades and his vision, shared by many others, that a very substantial reduction in the prevalence and severity of arteriosclerosis is possible from dietary supplementation alone. Large-scale studies currently underway suggest they are correct. We feel a future based on the findings of these scientists and their implementation through diet will substantially lower cardiovascular disease and the need for medication. Diet and proper nutrition also holds the promise for reversing the rising tide of Type 2 diabetes in adults, a tide that is now also afflicting young children. The problem is becoming so acute in the West and in some Asian developing countries that doctors consider being grossly overweight and the high risk of contracting diabetes to be intimately connected. So much so that a new term "diabesity," a blend of "diabetes" and "obesity," has been coined to sum up the escalating problem.

Elevated cholesterol is not the problem we have been led to believe. Yes it is a component of atherosclerotic plaque but a passive one. As McCully has stated, our present emphasis on cholesterol control requires dispassionate

125

reassessment. Based on the myriad problems associated with low cholesterol levels that we have reported, some would state that low cholesterol is more of a problem than high cholesterol. A decade ago such a statement would have clearly been a joke, but today the research evidence gives compelling support to its truth.

Just as McCully's work has been very influential in our research for this book, so can it be a vital resource for the many health organizations in our country that are involved in making dietary decisions. We need new dietary guidelines for the public and the food industry. We need to get back to basics in the field of nutrition. There is reason to believe that a national diet more liberal in protein and certain natural fats and far more restrictive in refined (or any) carbohydrates would be a major step forward. A number of excellent dietary guidelines of this type are available but Dr. McCully's Heart Revolution Diet[6] is given special consideration in this book because of its focus on homocysteine and nutritional deficiencies as the etiologic agents in arteriosclerosis.

And, finally, now knowing cholesterol's critical role in brain function and statins' drug's almost inevitable tendency for serious side effects, I am incredulous that statin drugs are proposed so liberally. So much of what we are, biochemically, is so completely dependent upon the so-called HMG-COA reductase process - the point of attack of the statin drugs and the target of the pharmaceutical industry in their zeal for cholesterol control. Our very life is threatened by disruption of the process at this point.

The present trend toward broader and broader use of statin drugs must be re-evaluated in light of the very compelling evidence that lowering cholesterol is not the solution to lowering the devastating effects of arteriosclerosis. There is no better time than now to challenge this national usage trend. The statin drugs are not without risk. Certainly the many deaths from rhabdomyolysis clearly point to serious and unpredictable risk. And these deaths are still occurring, despite the FDA's belated recall of Baycol®. The cognitive side effects such as amnesia and memory loss are of particular interest, not only because of the many cases already reported but also for those cases that will never be reported because they are too subtle. They are lost forever in that wasteland of forgotten things in the mind, mistakenly presumed to be part of our heritage of imprecision and the best our memories can do. In other words, it is likely that the reported cognitive events are but the tip of the iceberg in regard to the true incidence of statin "costs." Our memory is so important to us that any hint of threat, particularly from drugs that were prescribed for a totally unrelated medical condition, strikes at the very core of our being.

"What other recourse do we have?" ask the cardiologists and the primary care physicians, beleaguered by the pharmaceutical industry, the dictates of organized medicine, peer pressure and patient demands and fueled by direct-to-patient advertising. "Statins are all we have."

Lee of the Thrombosis and Vascular Biology Unit of Birmingham's City Hospital in the U.K. would say omega-3 and he brilliantly presents his documentation[7]. There is no longer any doubt as to the vital role of this polyunsaturated fatty acid in reducing cardiovascular disease risk. Not only has it been firmly documented to stabilize the myocardium electrically, resulting in reduced ventricular arrhythmias and sudden death but also it has been found to have potent anti-inflammatory effects quite comparable to those of the statin drugs. Robust supplementation of omega-3 via fish oils or other sources is strongly recommended.

Coenzyme Q10 say the Langsjoens in their overview of the use of coenzyme Q10 in cardiovascular disease[8] and word of the now indisputable adverse effect of statin drugs on our heart's mitochondrial function is slowly and reluctantly being admitted by the medical establishment. Statin drugs are now well known to severely inhibit our CoQ10 stores and our prevailing diet is such that our only recourse is robust supplementation, especially if one is on a statin.

The benefits of vitamin E and magnesium are referenced by Kauffman in his review of aspirin compared with other modalities for both primary and secondary prevention of cardiovascular disease.[9] Kauffman cites the special effectiveness of Bufferin because the magnesium benefit of the enteric coating supplements the established benefit of low-dose aspirin. Generally speaking, low dose "baby" 81 mg suffices and evidence is growing that it is of far greater benefit in secondary prevention, "after the MI" than primary, "before the MI".

Lower homocysteine would be the advice of Kilmer McCully, stressing the prevalence of subtle deficiencies of Vitamins B6 and B12 and folic acid in our over-nourished society. There is no longer any doubt as to the validity of McCully's position and whether a patient has a genetically preordained homocysteine elevation or the surprisingly prevalent acquired inability to take in sufficient daily amounts of these vital substances or simply doesn't know, these supplements are safe, economical and effective. McCully generally recommends 80-100mg of B6, 200-250mcg of B12 and 400-800mcg of folic acid daily.

The drug companies say, "Use our statins," with decreasing regard for cholesterol levels and increasing emphasis on the newly recognized anti-inflammatory action of these drugs. If statins are a super-aspirin it must be so stated. Promotional literature must turn away from current emphasis on cholesterol control for that does not appear to be our problem, arteriosclerosis control is, and inflammation of arterial linings is a well-documented factor in plaque formation. A super-aspirin is needed but one with an acceptable side effect profile. The side effects of current statin drugs seriously limit justification of use for primary prevention. Much more developmental work is necessary to perfect a suitable class of drugs for this purpose.

No discussion of statin drug use and cholesterol control would be complete without special consideration given to familial hypercholesterolemia (FH). Patients with grossly elevated serum cholesterols, with and without triglyceride levels in the thousands are a particular challenge to every primary care physician. For many of the unfortunate patients now bearing this genetic mandate the family history is replete with tragically early demise from cardiovascular complications yet others, with identical genetic patterns, lead long and healthy lives, strongly suggesting the presence of other factors of an environmental nature. Another curious observation from family tree mortality data[10] is that specific disease mortality among persons with FH living back in the mid to late 19th century differed little if at all from those free of FH then. Despite grossly elevated cholesterol and triglyceride patterns, longevity was unchanged for the great majority of those afflicted with FH. Scientists have inferred from this that elevated serum lipids may have afforded special protection from infectious disease, the big killer in those days. But mortality for those with FH rose after 1920, peaking around 1960 to its present level. Our FH cases, then, have shown a pattern of specific mortality similar to our general population but still with that very inconsistent finding of premature death from heart attacks and strokes for many but normal longevity for others. There seems little doubt that for this sub-group of patients, the presence of elevated lipids profoundly accelerates the inflammatory process underlying their arteriosclerosis and atherosclerosis. Such patients must be treated aggressively with every treatment option we have. The focus of attention should be directed primarily at underlying arterial inflammation and not solely on lipid control. Moderate doses of statins for their anti-inflammatory effect, supplemented by liberal omega 3, vitamins B6, B12 and folic acid, Coenzyme Q10, anti-oxidants and a daily 81mg Bufferin (for both magnesium and ASA) all should be considered as part of the treatment plan for this very high-risk patient group.

Studies that explore the use of statin drugs for stroke and heart attack prevention have yielded extraordinarily inconsistent findings. The truly comprehensive study conducted by Dr. Collins[11] of Oxford University proved that his heart patients lowered their risk of heart attacks and strokes by one-third after taking statins. On the basis of such seemingly positive findings, Dr. Collins estimates that an additional 200 million persons worldwide could benefit from this drug that he considers the "new aspirin" for warding off heart trouble.

Yet, Dr. Joel M. Kauffman, reporting on a long-term study by Jackson, et al[12] finds that long-term use of statins for primary prevention of heart disease produced a 1 percent greater risk of death over 10 years vs. placebo when the results of all the big controlled trials reported before 2000 were combined. Dr. Kauffman noted further that even for short-term use, 16 weeks in the MIRACL study by Schwartz, et al[13], in patients with heart or angina problems, the use of Lipitor® (atorvastatin) at a rich 80 mg/day did not significantly change the all cause death rate or the rate of heart attacks. Such inconsistencies naturally make interpretation of these kinds of data extremely difficult and underscores the crucial need for the members of the pharmaceutical industry to make patient safety their priority, since side effects are probable and benefit is not.

That the cognitive and behavioral side effect problems of the statin drugs are just being recognized in the utilization of these drugs is a direct result of the current flawed research and disinformation processes of the pharmaceutical companies. The incomplete and misleading information currently being distributed to doctors and patients as a result of those flawed processes has created a vacuum of awareness of the potential memory problems even as it almost guarantees an enormous profit return. In fact, in 2003, Pfizer's Lipitor® became the first $10 billion drug in history[14]. (Fortune® article)

The FDA must initiate, with congressional support, a complete revamping and revitalization of its policies for approval and distribution of the pharmaceutical industry's drugs and products. This initiative must define patient safety as the primary reason for the FDA's very existence. It must also resist any and all industry efforts to fast track their medications for approval in order to insure that company's market share. It should request and welcome the establishment of an independent National Medications Safety Board, funded by the pharmaceutical industry, to oversee the safety of post-approval medications and all other aspects of the drug industry.

Even more importantly, the pharmaceutical industry must be compelled to conform to the same high ethics in the production and marketing of their products that physicians are held to. They need to be made aware of the consequences of their pursuit for exorbitant market and profit return at the cost of mounting loss of patient and doctor confidence. The extraordinarily high pedestal most patients place their doctors on deserves that equally high standards are defined and maintained for the medications those doctors dispense. The annual toll of lives and serious side effects currently sustained by hundreds of thousands of patients is a heavy and unnecessary price to pay for faith misplaced.

And looming large in the near future is the very real possibility of "pay back" time for the pharmaceutical companies. The current class action law suits being tried in American courts as a result of the statin drug, Baycol®, and its lethal side effects in the death of dozens of patients and the many recent filings of Lipitor® damage claims appear to be just the beginning. Those hidden side effects of Baycol® before the FDA finally recalled it are being noted by some of the nation's top plaintiff's attorneys as they train their sites on the drug industry. After successfully fighting the asbestos and tobacco companies, these attorneys are ready to claim that many giant pharmaceutical companies, in hiding the dangers of their medicines, have harmed thousands of people.

An indisputable, ironic double loss occurs when half of the patients in this country discontinue urgently needed medications because of preventable side effects. "The patient loses by becoming exposed to markedly increased risks of premature disease and death," advises Dr. Jay Cohen[15], and the drug industry loses increased drug sales when patients become dissatisfied with a medication and discontinue treatment.

The attending physician, the patient and the drug industry all lose when drug side effects are unacceptable. This irony is particularly true when these side effects include the theft of our most precious commodity, our very memory.

In the last decade mankind received an incredible research result - the gift of DNA mapping, which introduces wave after wave of astonishing new information promising us the ability to tailor a drug to a patient's specific needs based upon his or her genome. The reality is that this incredible feat is already here and will soon be commonplace. Not only will we be able to predict with complete confidence which of our available drugs are most effective for a patient's specific needs, but we also will be able to choose the drug least likely to have serious side effects. DNAPrint® Genomics[11] is already offering a service known as

Statnome to help better match the statin drug to the patient and this is just the beginning.

Specific DNA printing is in the very near future, but in today's world, with our ability to predict side effects still in an almost primitive state; we allow much too liberal statin drug use. As the zeal for primary prevention by both the pharmaceutical industry and organized medicine serve to promote wider and wider utilization of these powerful drugs, harmful side effects become an immediate concern. The physiological implications of these drugs are profound when based on just what is actually known at this time, but when one adds the reality of our present shallow grasp of physiology at the intracellular and molecular level, there is justification for the question, "Do we really know what we are doing?"

ADDENDUM

This somewhat more technical part of the book dealing with the neurophysiologic mechanisms defining special susceptibility to statins, mechanisms of cognitive impairment from statins, effects of statins on sexuality and the unusual association of statin therapy to such neuro-degenerative diseases as ALS, Parkinsonism and frontal lobe dementia was prepared specifically for practicing physicians to aid in their management of these often obscure conditions. The lay reader may find much of this information difficult to assimilate but the cardiovascular risk determination and sexuality aspects are appropriate for both lay and professional readers. I recommend that all lay readers at least scan this material.

a. Genetic Susceptibility and Abnormal Pathways of Statin Drugs' Effect.

Now we suspect that some patients may have a genetic susceptibility to statin–induced problems. Special genetic susceptibility may explain not only much of our statin associated rhabdomyolysis but also the curious pattern of persistent myopathy and the recent observation of post polio syndrome aggravation, often following only a short course of statins. Since susceptibility testing of this type is not yet widely available, there is no practical way to identify these susceptibles until the damage is done.

One of these genetically determined enzymatic conditions is carnitine palmitoyl transferase (CPT) deficiency[1]. The enzymes involved are found on different membranes of our mitochondria, those busy factories within each of our cells responsible for the production of our (ATP) energy. Produced in each of our body's million's of cells, mitochondrial ATP is our body's sole source of energy. CPT enzymes work together with Coenzyme Q10 in the process of transport of fatty acids into our mitochondria and their ultimate conversion into fuel. Deficiency of this class of enzymes is characterized by unusual muscle pain and stiffness after exercise or work.

Certain types of muscle cells are especially dependant upon carnitine for fatty acid transport. CoQ10 also helps in this complex metabolic interplay. When these substances are insufficient, myopathy may result. This is particularly true in those having unusual CPT molecular mutations. Especially under conditions of CoQ10 deficiency such as that known to occur with the use of statin drugs, this persistent type of myopathy may result.

One can hardly justify the statin class of drugs for wide-scale use as in primary prevention and over the counter distribution (as in Britain) when the completely unpredictable end-point may be rhabdomyolysis death, initiation of post polio syndrome or permanent myopathic debility.

Another novel mechanism of action for statin side effects on the Golgi apparatus was recently reported. The Golgi apparatus, along with a tubular network called the endoplasmic reticulum, is present in every cell in our body, controlling vital cell interactions. Now our scientists are just beginning to reveal the actual mechanics of cholesterol's role in statin associated behavioral change – another pathway not yet dreamed of only a year ago. Reporting in Science recently Wang and Anderson[2] have discovered a critical role for cell cholesterol in the Golgi apparatus role of cell signaling. They found that oxysterol binding protein (OSBP) is a cholesterol-binding "scaffolding" protein vital to the control of signaling pathways within the Golgi apparatus. These researchers found this vital pathway extremely sensitive to cholesterol levels within the cells. When intracellular cholesterol was lowered by whatever means, profound degradation of this signaling pathway resulted

On another front, Meske[3] found in his neuron cell cultures that blocking the usual cholesterol dependent pathway with lovastatin (Mevacor) evoked not only degeneration of the neuritic network of the neurons under study but also a transient increase of tau phosphorylation.

To refresh your memory, tau is that protein so prominently deposited in the brains in Alzheimers patients and also has been observed in other of our neuro-degenerative diseases. These abnormally phosphorulated tau proteins may go on to form the neurofibrillatory tangles seen in amyotrophic lateral sclerosis, progressive surpanuclear palsy, multiple system atrophy, fronto-temporal dementia, cortico-basilar degeneration and selected cases of Parkinson's disease. While blocking cholesterol, statins appear to block our more natural mevalonate pathways resulting in activation of abnormal tau phosphorylation. The result of this is increased deposition of tau protein leading to increased neuronal degeneration in the presence of beta-amyloid. In the absence of tau protein these neurons did not degenerate. These findings underscore both the importance of tau protein in the pathogenesis of Alzheimers and the apparent enhancement of tau deposition by statin drug use. Despite reports to the contrary, it would seem that a major effect of statin on Alzheimers is one of aggravating the underlying condition. Any reported benefit of statins on this condition must derive from statins' inherent anti-inflammatory effect, for Alzheimers has a definite inflammatory component. Meanwhile the underlying pathology, the reason for the inflammation in the first place, may well be aggravated.

Another recently reported novel pathway for statin associated myopathy has recently been reported by Chapman and Carrie[4]. Their work on the ubiquitin proteasome pathway (UPP) shows a possible effect of statin drugs on this mechanism to explain myopathy. In one unpublished study, although the combination of statin and rest had little effect on gene expression, when exercise was added, multiple genes were differentially expressed of which 18% involved the UPP and 20% involved protein folding and catabolism and apopotosis. The analysis of data thus far suggests that, "statins may alter the response of muscle to exercise stress by altering the action of the UPP, protein folding, and catabolism, disrupting the balance between protein degradation and repair."

To translate this largely incomprehensible extract of that paper, "statins interfere with muscle action". I admit that reading the above is tough going for a layperson and it is tough going for a medical doctor. I cite this evolving research area only to document the existence of these alternative means by which statin drugs can cause such diverse side effects in susceptible individuals. We are just beginning to understand these effects!

b. What is your Cardiovascular Risk?

Only a short time ago one's cardiovascular disease risk was defined primarily by the cholesterol level, giving demerits for obesity, couch potato tendencies, and smoking but focusing on one's cholesterol level, so easily measured and potentially controllable with pharmaceuticals. Starting four decades ago, guided by the grossly manipulated dietary studies of the crafty Ancel Keys, we began our ride on the cholesterol bandwagon. Any doctor not in tune with this new cholesterol music was grossly uninformed or hopelessly ignorant. For every 1% our serum cholesterol could be lowered, we were promised a 2% reduction in our cardiovascular risk. Following my internship, I joined thousands of other young, fellow doctors in writing prescriptions for whatever cholesterol buster the pharmaceutical industry was promoting at the time. We talked at service clubs and libraries and to our incredulous patients of the newly recognized dangers of whole milk, eggs and butter. The low fat, low cholesterol diet was in. We lauded the arrival of, our first really effective cholesterol lowering medication, the statin drugs. The food industry long ago joined the drug companies in the fight against cholesterol, for billions of dollars were to be made in the manufacture of specially prepared foodstuffs for our supermarket shelves. This was a win-win situation for everybody. The drug and food industry were making billions, the medical community was busier than ever and our patients had high hopes of snatching years of useful life from the grim reaper. Think of this as the Titanic in motion, think of the immense inertia of the prevailing system.

Now, in the past year or so, our longitudinal studies have revealed an amazing truth. Cholesterol is not the cause of increased cardiovascular risk with its atherosclerosis and strokes, inflammation is. Abruptly it was learned that statins have their remarkable ability to lower one's cardiovascular risk not because of cholesterol manipulation but by an inherent, and previously unsuspected, anti-inflammatory effect. Cholesterol is once again recognized for what it was forty years ago – the most important biochemical in our bodies. Without abundant cholesterol neither our brain nor our bodies can function properly. Whoops, say our national leaders in diet and health, the cholesterol bandwagon was misguided. It is back now to eggs, butter and whole milk. Meanwhile the Titanic still forges ahead, the habits of forty years hard for doctors to break, especially with the pharmaceutical industry still valiantly trying to preserve the still lucrative market for their highly profitable cash cows. Is it any wonder patients are confused?

If cholesterol doesn't matter any more what is your cardiovascular risk? In reality the strongest determinant of cardiovascular risk is your personal and family history. If your blood relatives experienced premature heart attacks and strokes, you are high risk, regardless of your cholesterol level, even if it is less than 100. Similarly, if you have experienced a transient ischemic attack (TIA) or were found to have a silent myocardial infarction (MI) on routine electrocardiogram, you are high risk, regardless of your cholesterol level. Gross obesity, high blood pressure, sedentary life style and cigarette smoking all predispose you to cardiovascular disease but your history is a far more definitive marker. In medicine, as in so many other things in life, there are few absolutes so even a "bad" history can be mellowed by life style changes.

True, your CRP level is an inflammatory marker, but even with its more recent refinements in specificity, it remains only a very gross indicator of underlying arterial wall inflammation. All too often an elevated value reflects a completely unrelated inflammatory process. We must remember that a large number of conditions, including sinusitis, periodontal disease, apical abscess, bronchitis, cholecystitis, cystitis, urethritis, prostatitis and pelvic infection may be low grade, without significant symptoms. Any of these often, obscure conditions may result in elevations of CRP and be a frustratingly common source of false positives regarding screening for arterial inflammation.

Another marker of only general significance may be your homocysteine level. True, high levels of homocysteine are very closely associated with cardiovascular disease risk. This relationship has been demonstrated in numerous studies, yet there is some reason to suspect that homocysteine may be a far better marker of past arterial disease rather than present. Finding an elevated homocysteine level in someone known to have sustained a stroke or heart attack, then lowering homocysteine in this same individual by aggressive vitamin B6, 12 or folic acid supplementation does not give impressive lowering of cardiovascular risk of future episodes. Obviously this implies that low homocysteine may exert its benefit early on in primary prevention before the onset of disease rather than in secondary prevention, although proof of this hypothesis remains to be determined.

Another substance having significant potential as a screening tool for high cardiovascular risk is lipoprotein (a)[1]. For 40 million years we primates have relied on the atherogenic potential of lipoprotein (a) to protect us from "tooth and claw". We traded our ability to synthesize vitamin C for the hemostatic benefit of lipoprotein (a) because this chance mutation, almost certainly cosmic radiation induced, gave a definite survival advantage as our ancestors emerged from the trees. Now, we (with only our fellow primates and guinea pigs) are the only mammals bearing our present, unusual predisposition to atherosclerosis. If lipoprotein (a) is found to be unusually elevated, one always has recourse to vitamin C with or without supplemental proline and lysine. Lipoprotein (a) has not yet been widely accepted as the marker it is but in my judgment it has much potential in preventive medicine.

On the this subject of disease screening and markers we must remember that DNA mapping, unheard of a few years ago, now is about to lead us into the future of clinical medicine. In the last decade mankind has received this incredible gift. Each day sees wave after wave of astonishing new DNA mapping information promising us the ability not only to detect with astonishing accuracy the genetically pre-ordained disease timeline of an individual but also the ability to tailor a treatment plan specific to a patient's needs. The reality is that this incredible feat is already here and will soon be commonplace. Not only will we be able to predict with complete confidence which therapies are most effective for a patient's specific needs, but also will be able to choose a treatment least likely to have serious side effects. Specific DNA printing with its promise of dramatic change in health care delivery is very nearly here.

In today's world, with our ability to predict needs and sensitivities still in an almost primitive state, we allow much too liberal statin drug use. I well remember the words of Doctor Elsworth

Amidon, professor of medicine during my medical school days, "Every new drug you give to your patient is the start of an experiment." The more we learn about our DNA, which varies so dramatically from that of our fellow man, the more we realize this statement is true. To give a genetically predisposed patient a statin may well trigger fatal rhabdomyolysis or permanent myopathy. Rare, perhaps, but to the patient, if he or she lives, your competence as a doctor has taken a new low. As the zeal for primary prevention by both the pharmaceutical industry and organized medicine strives to promote higher doses and wider utilization of these powerful drugs, harmful side effects will become an even greater problem than we face today. The physiological implications of these drugs are profound when based on just what is actually known at this time, but when one adds the reality of our present shallow grasp of physiology at the intracellular level, there is justification for the question, "Do we really know what we are doing?"

Until we get DNA mapping, the most accurate marker of cardiovascular risk is personal and family history (which, of course, are genetically based). Serum levels of homocysteine and lipoprotein (a) may give useful supplemental information. The CRP, if negative (or very low) is a useful marker of inflammation. High values are often misleading due to the inherent non-specificity of this test. Far better markers of inflammation at the endothelial level are indicated.

c. Mechanisms of Transient Global Amnesia

Transient global amnesia is not new, nor is it a medical malady that has 'arrived' recently due to increasingly sophisticated medical diagnostic ability. For nearly fifty years researchers have been attempting to discover the underlying cause. Today, despite the availability of imaging technology not even dreamed of five decades ago, lack of agreement still exists as to the precise factors involved. Each of the several possible mechanisms has had its share of ardent and strong-willed advocates. Many firmly believe that the vasospastic etiology of migraine explains it all, by pointing to the large numbers of cases where various imaging techniques have revealed indisputable evidence of diminished blood flow in those areas of the brain known to be involved in memory processing and retrieval. Others, at one time or another, have pointed to epilepsy as the trigger mechanism, offering various explanations as to why the EEGs in classic global amnesia cases are consistently free of epileptiform activity. Admittedly, the well-known amnesic aura of epilepsy comes extraordinarily close in clinical presentation to classic transient global amnesia. Still others point to cerebrovascular factors comparable to those causing transient ischemic attacks as responsible. If so, the cause might be a loose cluster of platelets cells clinging together sufficiently long to transiently block circulation before breaking up and reverting to normal blood flow. Closely related to this is the possibility that venous congestion may be contributory. Lewis[1] has proposed that venous congestion, by causing disruption of blood flow to key brain structures, may help explain the unusual association of strenuous exercise, highly active sex, cold water immersion, and the Valsalva maneuver with transient global amnesia attacks. For similar reasons others have suggested that whatever elevates intrathoracic pressure inevitably contributes to venous congestion with its possible sequellae.

This would appear to be the logical place to discuss physical and biological factors: patent foramen ovale. Most readers have never heard of this vital structure that is the source of our ability to live while completely immersed in liquid. Throughout the nine months we float about in the amniotic fluid of our mother's uterus, breathing in the normal sense is impossible. Our lungs have no function in this environment. Mother Nature benevolently decreed we should bypass the lungs during our "underwater" gestation.

Venous blood entering the right atrium of the heart is diverted from the lungs directly into the comparable chamber on the left side of the heart, through our patent foramen ovale. This subject of circulation of blood in the fetus is a fascinating one but, other than for the foramen ovale, not relevant to the subject of transient global amnesia. What is relevant, however, is the astonishing frequency wherein this life-giving opening fails to close securely after our first few breaths, when it no longer is needed. This subject has intrigued researchers in the field of cerebrovascular accidents and Homma[2] reports that approximately 40 per cent of cerebral infarctions that cannot be classified as strokes of determined cause, despite a complete diagnostic work-up, are labeled as "cryptogenic strokes." Contrast echocardiography in such patients has revealed an extremely high incidence of patent foramen ovale, with values as high as 40 percent. Of particular interest are the values ranging from 20 to 55 percent for transient global amnesia patients. Precise data on the incidence of this finding in the general public are difficult to obtain but it has been estimated to be as high as 10 percent.

The incidence of this abnormality has come to light only in the past several decades, as imaging technology has become both more precise and available. But the impact is a sobering awareness that many of us have patent foramen ovale and, with it, the potential for the same right to left shunting of blood that made our fetal lives possible. The problem is that as adults we carry the risk that emboli of one type of another can now pass directly into our brains. We have lost the "safety net" of having our venous blood thoroughly filtered by our lungs.

So far, none of this would seem to have any bearing on the effect of statin drugs on memory and other cognitive functions, but since there are two sides to every coin, there is an opposite side to this right-to-left shunt that is very relevant. To have this right to left shunt presupposes that on occasion the pressure within the right atrial chamber exceeds that of the left. When this point is reached, venous blood, platelet emboli, nitrogen bubbles or "what have you" pass over to their destiny on the left side of the body. Anything that raises venous pressure, be it vigorous sex, strenuous exercise, performing the Valsalva maneuver for your doctor, positive pressure breathing with a mask as in diving and high altitude vacuum chambers, or in vigorous coughing- -the possibilities are many - produces the same results. But what of the other times, when you are resting? This is when you have the left to right shunt because the pressure on the left ordinarily greatly exceeds the right. The shunt of blood may not be much, perhaps just a few cubic centimeters every heartbeat, but it is still easily enough to raise venous pressure above normal and keep it there. The result is venous congestion, creating potential interference with blood flow and tissue metabolism upstream, which is analogous to building a dam across a stream with predictable consequences to the flow of water. Lewis's interesting concept of venous pressure as a trigger to transient global amnesia becomes much more interesting when one considers the reality that many of us may have patent foramen ovale.

Since we are on the subject of plumbing variations and their not so subtle effects on circulation, what of the well-known subclavian steal syndrome? Using the old adage of "robbing Peter to pay Paul," we can simplify the explanation. With society's awareness of the DNA mandated differences that make each of us so unique, it is not surprising to learn of the many different ways arterial blood is carried to our heads and brain. In many of us the right vertebral artery branches from our subclavian artery rather than directly from the aorta. As some of you know, our subclavian artery supplies our arm (Paul) and our vertebral artery connects with other arteries in the brain (Peter). The steal part occurs when vigorous arm activity demands more blood than the subclavian can supply from its origin at the aorta. It then 'steals'" from the vertebral, depriving the brain of sufficient blood and oxygen during the arm exercise. This becomes particularly interesting when one learns that the stolen blood was originally intended to supply brain tissue involved in memory. Whether from diminished arterial flow or congestion of venous return from increased pressure, the ischemic results on the tissues involved can be quite comparable.

Only one other possibility of any merit remains - spreading depression, a condition that is described by some as the electrochemical equivalent of surgical ablation. Once triggered, this deactivation process slowly sweeps across the involved area of brain tissue causing oxygen and glucose uptake to all but cease while creating a sharp rise of extracellular potassium and precipitous falls of both sodium and chloride. From the viewpoint of a cell this is serious business, indeed, for the energy of a cell is completely dependent upon the balance of these ions. Potassium ions on the outside of a cell wall are like an uncharged battery. We are dealing with a slowly spreading area of tissue depleted of the very stuff of life. Then, into this all but dead zone of brain tissue flows a massive influx of calcium and the condition rapidly can become a life or death matter. Fortunately, recovery is the rule where the trigger agent is transient, and the body slowly reverses the process. Those studying animal models of stroke can control whether or not tissue death will occur simply by juggling the acidity levels and the balance of these ions.

Fortunately, in our classic transient global amnesia cases, Mother Nature remains firmly in control. A vasospastic insult or a fleeting thromboembolic one may trigger spreading depression, preventing for a time the laying down of new memories or recovery of past ones, but it remains transitory, resolving within twenty-four hours. This proposed mechanism for transient global amnesia is rapidly gaining acceptance as research data present an ever more convincing case. Interestingly, this process closely resembles the much more serious sequence of events seen in stroke, either ischemic or hemorrhagic. The end result is ischemia of brain tissue, triggering spreading depression. Whether recovery or death ensues depends entirely on the degree and duration of ischemia.

Migraine is a class of recurrent headaches so common that nearly everyone has heard of them. Occasionally the headache is preceded by an "aura." The aura typically involves visual changes, such as seeing wavy lines, spots or even hallucinations.

Auras have been consistently tied to a phenomenon known as cortical spreading depression, during which a wave of altered brain activity sweeps across the cortex of the brain. Frank Richter,[3] reported on the failure of cortical spreading depression to fully explain migraine headache, despite offering a firm neurophysiological basis for aura. This would seem to be a process similar, if not identical to, the spreading depression process just described, with the difference being primarily one of location in the brain. If located in the memory structures of the brain, transient global amnesia may result; if the occipital cortex is involved, the auras of migraine follow.

Yes, transient global amnesia is related to migraines and there seems to be some crossing over of neurophysiology but they are different. Only a relatively small percentage of transient global amnesia patients have a migraine history and the triggers, especially the venous pressure feature, are noticeably lacking in migraine.

Returning to the transient global amnesia syndrome and the similarity of signs and symptoms that herald the likely diagnosis to the experienced examiner: why are patients so much alike despite the disparity in age, gender and precipitating factors? The answer would seem to be the final common pathway concept mentioned earlier. The diverse nature of precipitating factors seems to condense to very small numbers when the venous congestion concept is considered. Ischemia of certain of the tissues involved in memory could be the final insult that initiates the potentially harmful spreading depression. It is relevant to consider how the statins fit this paradigm.

Since, as Pfrieger[4] has proven, biosynthesis of cholesterol at the glial cell is imperative for neuronal function and synapse formation, the statin drugs, the HMG-CoA reductase inhibitors, sensitize us, in a manner of speaking, to the slightest hint of altered brain metabolism. Transient spreading depression tolerable to many as nothing or a minor nuisance well might be magnified in those in whom neuronal tissue is under the effect of statins. As one hovers on the edge of synaptic competence due to statin drug effect, the slightest hint of impairment of neuronal glucose, or oxygen consumption, or altered ionic balance such as might ensue with spreading depression, might be just sufficient to tilt a patient toward transient global amnesia.

At the time of this writing, spreading depression remains the 'best fit' mechanism to explain the "final neurophysiologic pathway" of transient global amnesia. It offers a framework within which one can explain either the milder cases wherein the presenting deficit is primarily anterograde amnesia, or the much more complex cases where both anterograde and retrograde amnesia to the patient's distant past occur. It also offers an explanation for the permanent obliteration of memory occasionally seen, and even for those cases in which several days may be required for recovery. As to trigger factors, venous congestion has definite physiological appeal and certainly fits the observed data quite well. When one considers the added predisposition of those among us with hidden patent foramen ovale or susceptibility to subclavian steal, venous congestion becomes particularly congruous.

Obviously, not all factors hang so comfortably on our venous congestion/spreading depression framework. What of the "traveler's amnesia" associated with benzodiazapine use? Can this be considered the same as transient global amnesia? Most regard its lack of repetitive questioning and exclusively anterograde qualities as evidence that it is not. The majority considers the altered memory, occasional depersonalization, confusion, and hallucinations as evidence of a central nervous system depressant activity. We must leave the final determination on this to future research.

The quite common association of transient global amnesia with cerebral angiography deserves another question mark as to mechanism. Are tiny emboli released into the carotid artery, secondary to the process of catheter insertion or is the generally alien nature of the solution - definitely not your normal tissue perfusing solution - triggering a sort of mechanical embolization and transiently altering tissue metabolism; or is it a toxic reaction in certain individuals? Any of these choices might conceivably serve to trigger a spreading reaction but at this point must remain conjecture.

d. Statins and Sexuality

The pharmaceutical industry would lead us to believe that rapidly bottoming out our natural cholesterol levels through the use of their highly touted statin drugs is a relatively innocuous process of definite benefit to society. But as we learn more each day of this ubiquitous and unique cholesterol substance, we must question the veracity of their medical advisors. Cholesterol is perhaps the most important substance in our lives for we could not live without an abundant supply of it in our bodies.

Researchers everywhere are learning how extraordinarily complex and often surprising are the pathways that produce and metabolize cholesterol. Cholesterol is the precursor for a whole class of hormones known as the steroid hormones that are absolutely critical for life, as we know it. These hormones determine our sexuality, control the reproductive process, and regulate blood sugar levels and mineral metabolism. This same substance that society has been taught to fear happens to be our sole source for our sex hormones, androgen, estrogen and progesterone. Researchers marvel at the remarkable similarity in chemical structure these sex hormones have with each other and with the original cholesterol parent from which they are derived. One might say the glaring family resemblance attests to the mighty power of a methyl group here and a carboxyl group there. The destiny of us all is marvelously controlled by such seemingly minor changes. Now with our much-

155

touted statin drugs we are reducing the bio-availability of our natural cholesterol to levels never before seen in large population groups. Since cholesterol is the basis of the vital hormones controlling our sexuality, one can logically expect sexuality problems if this precursor substance becomes sufficiently lowered. The question is, "Do our statin drugs as currently used adversely affect sexuality?"

Anecdotal reports have been surfacing for years of impotence, loss of libido and erectile dysfunction associated with statin drug use. I have summarized the available review articles, called attention to the most relevant of anecdotal case reports, reviewed relevant research studies and included a list of most relevant references in the preparation of this paper.

The findings of Kash Rizvi[1] et al in their 2002 review of erectile dysfunction leave little doubt that a strong relationship exists between the taking of statin drugs and erectile dysfunction. Applying the criteria suggested by Sackett and colleagues in their book, "Clinical Epidemiology: A Basic Science for Clinical Medicine" most would say that the strength of the relationship is sufficiently strong that it should be called "probably causal". This comes regardless of the indefinite nature of the many factors contributing to erectile dysfunction and impotence such as the psychologic influences in a post-myocardial infarction situation, co-existing medical conditions and the well-known tendency for under-reporting and possible contributions from other medications known to be possibly contributory. It is not an easy subject to investigate. They reported 42 cases of erectile dysfunction associated with simvastatin in an Australian study[2] with four having recurrence with rechallenge. As might be expected, the strongest factor in proving causality has been recurrence of the problem with statin rechallenge.

In a review of France and Spain's adverse drug reports by Bagheri and others[3], 74 cases of impotence associated with statin drug use were reported. In 85% of these cases the condition regressed completely when the statin drug was stopped. Six of the French cases reported return of symptoms with rechallenge. The others presumably "passed" on the offer to retake the statin. This review failed to find a significant difference between statins in regards to impotence frequency.

Bruckert[4] et al concluded that erectile dysfunction is a frequent disorder in hyperlipidemic men treated with statins and/or fibric acid derivatives. Their study group consisted of 339 age-matched men 40-50 years of age. If these otherwise healthy men were on a statin drug, impotence was much more likely.

L. de Graff[5] and colleagues reported that decreased libido is a probable adverse drug reaction of statin drugs and is generally reversible. They added that this reaction may be caused by low serum testosterone levels, mainly due to cholesterol depletion. They reported two cases of low libido during statin drug use in which low serum testosterone levels returned to normal levels after the statin drug was discontinued.

Jackson[6] reported on five men with coronary artery disease who developed impotence within one week of starting treatment with simvastatin 10 mg or having the dose increased to 20 mg. Within one week of stopping simvastatin, sexual function was restored. Two patients were rechallenged with simvastatin and impotence recurred. Jackson suggested that simvastatin might affect the central nervous system directly by passing through the blood-brain-barrier.

All investigators in this field stress the likelihood of gross under-reporting of impotence, erectile dysfunction and loss of libido in the usual doctor/patient interaction. If the examining physician does not specifically ask the question as to sexuality problems, it is very unlikely to be brought up by the patient. When studied as a separate issue, however, the preceding reports well document the importance of impotence, loss of libido and erectile dysfunction as a statin drug side effect. Although some postulate a CNS explanation for the effect of statins on sexuality, diminished testosterone production due to relative depletion by statins of its cholesterol precursor deserves serious consideration as a causative factor.

The question is, "Do our statin drugs as currently used contribute significantly to loss of libido and erectile dysfunction?" Since cholesterol is the substrate for some of our most vital hormones, including testosterone, progesterone and estrogen, one can logically expect sexuality problems if this precursor substance becomes sufficiently lowered. Now with our much-touted, ever more powerful statin drugs, we are reducing the bio-availability of our natural cholesterol to levels never before seen in large population groups. The glaring advertisements promoting our most recent addition to the stable of statin workhorses, Crestor, lauds its ability to impair cholesterol biosynthesis as much as 52%.

The operative word here is significant for many factors contribute to libido loss and erectile dysfunction. Other medications, aging, stress are but a few of these other factors but they relate across the board. Who is free from aging, stress and other medications? How do you measure scientifically the impact of statins of libido? Such studies have been done and more studies are underway. Yes, statins deplete testosterone. The results of these studies are in the medical literature and cited in the Physician Desk Reference in every medical doctor's library.

The following statement appears in the conclusion of many of these studies: Decreased libido is a probable adverse drug reaction of HMG-CoA-reductase-inhibitors and is reversible. This adverse drug report may be caused by low serum testosterone levels, mainly due to intracellular cholesterol depletion.

So testosterone levels are depleted by statins – so what? Drug company researchers are well aware that testosterone blood levels correlate poorly with sex drive. Every student of this area knows that a high serum testosterone may be associated with complete lack of sexual interest and a low level for this substance is not at all unusual in sexual "athletes". There is an extremely wide range of normal with respect to testosterone levels. The key according to drug company researchers and primary care MDs counseling E.D. and low libido patients, is how your current blood level for testosterone compares with what it used to be, twenty years ago and, of course, most of us do not have this on record. Bottom line – "There is a consistent tendency for decreased testosterone biosynthesis once statins have been started but testosterone correlates poorly with sexuality therefore you can feel comfortable about "losing it". Researchers have done their duty, the data is presented "honestly' (pharmaceutical tracks have been artfully covered) and as the patient takes his first statin pill his thought is that, "It can never happen to me." Oh yes, one other thing – this is not just a man thing.

e. Statins' Neurodegenerative Effects.

I have received correspondence from many people who, while taking statins, have developed symptoms sufficiently similar to other well established neurodegenerative diseases that their initial diagnosis was considered to be Multiple Sclerosis (MS), Amyotrophic Lateral Sclerosis (ALS), Parkinson's Disease (PD), Frontal Lobe Dementia (FLD), Alzheimer's Disease (AD), Multiple System Abnormalities (MSA) Polymalgia Rheumatica (PR) and even somatic mitochondrial mutations. The presumed mechanism of action of such cases have been statin induced cholesterol inhibition, ubiquinone depletion, some combination of the two or some other as yet un-identified link.

Please refer to the preceding section dealing with other statin side effect pathways, especially to Meske's work on abnormal tau protein phosphorylation associated with statin use[1]. The role of this abnormal tau protein in the formation of the neurofibrillatory tangles (NFTs) and the association of these statin induced NFTs with many of the neurodegenerative diseases mentioned above is under active investigation at this time. This mechanism of statin associated abnormal tau phosphorylation may help us understand the frequent association of statin drug intake with certain neuro-degenerative diseases[2,3]. Meske has established induction of tau protein phosphorylation by statins as a consequence of statin inhibitory effect on the usual mevalonate pathways. Again we are seeing gross evidence of statin drug's collateral damage to existing cellular chemistry just as we have noted with statins' inhibition of dolichol, CoQ10 and glial cell cholesterol synthesis. And, we observe, all from statins' effect on our mevalonate pathway, originally conceived to inhibit cholesterol synthesis.

As you will note from the following case reports, ALS and PD are commonly reported soon after statin are initiated. Until now we have had no convincing explanation. The knowledge of the formation of tau protein abnormalities associated with the effect of statin drugs on the mevalonate pathway has opened up promising new areas for exploration.

In some of these cases the symptoms have regressed after stopping of the statin drug lending credence to possible statin drug causation. In other cases various supplements have been utilized in addition to stopping the statin drug, with varying degrees of improvement in the clinical picture depending on the nature of the supplements and dosages.

Since there are no therapeutic guidelines for such cases, treatment plans have been largely intuitive. Other cases have gone on to the classical forms of these various neurodegenerative diseases despite cessation of the statin, provoking the question as to what role, if any, their previous statin might have played in "triggering" their illness.

The following are a few of the reports I have received from readers of my books and website relevant to the subject of neurodegenerative diseases and statin drug use. Just to peruse these tragic cases may possibly lead some readers to greater awareness of the true legacy of statins in some people and help physicians establish a diagnosis when possible statin causation may not have been considered. It might be of interest to the readers that several of these statin associated reactions were experienced personally by MDs.

"I have found out my creatinine kinase was 386 on March 31, 2005 and was taken off Lipitor. I asked for my old records and found that it was at 237 in February of 2004 when I had been taking Lipitor for 14 months (20mg per day). With all the research I have done, I feel this was the cause, however, my doctor said he does not know what is wrong with me. Multiple Sclerosis was ruled out but I have neuropathy from elbows to hands, lost fine motor skills and walk unsteady. I have weakness and loss of muscle in my hands. I fell down the stairs last week. I work a physical job, need my income and I am only 55 yrs old."

"We went in to see the Doctor this afternoon. As a concession to my on-going effort to confirm the diagnosis of this ostensible mitochondrial dysfunction of mine, my doctor has agreed to drop my statin dose to 5 mg/day after my next catheterization for its value at reducing arterial inflammation. Since I will be on Ticlid for several months thereafter and will have to have my blood

work tested every two weeks anyway we can monitor the effect of the diminished statin drug on my cholesterol levels and see if it reduces the effects of my morning 'fugue'."

"My father began taking Lipitor around May 2002. It was shortly after that time that I noticed some changes in him. Sometimes he'd start a story then lose his place and other things were happening that he'd forget. This past summer (July 04) after being on Lipitor for almost 18 months, my Mom watched as he paused in writing a check to pay a bill. This is something he has always done, manage/pay all household bills. He couldn't remember how to write out the long hand form of the amount of money. He also became very quiet. Normally, he's the life of the party and wanting to chat with everyone. Instead he became quiet and would sit by himself at parties or with my Mom. Usually he'd be the one that would be the 'social butterfly' and leave my Mom. After my Mom mentioned this to her chiropractor, she was given an article on some of the side effects of Lipitor (it was an article from Newsweek). After reading this article, my Mom insisted that my Dad's primary care stop his Lipitor. My father has undergone a CAT scan, and MRI which have proved to all be normal. He also had some cognitive testing done which ruled out Alzheimers. We met with a neurologist last week, who wanted to run more tests. During the appt. the neurologist mentioned he thought it might be Frontal Lobe Dementia. At that time, those were merely three words. Now after

researching online, I have discovered this horrible disease (Pick's disease) and there is no cure and no treatment. Frontal Lobe Dementia has the exact same outcome as Alzheimer's; the only difference is there is less known about it. We asked the neurologist if Lipitor could be the reason behind this. Without hesitation, his reply was No."

"I have Familial Hypercholesterolemia and an horrendous "bad" cholesterol level that has NEVER been reduced to a medically satisfactory level. I started taking statins as soon as they were an alternative to cholestyramine, which was disgusting to take. I have experienced just about all of the side effects that I have, fairly recently, discovered to be rampant among statin users. All of these effects were dismissed by my doctors, none of whom took the connection seriously. I suffered the most trouble when, after my first cardiac catheterization, my cardiologist increased my dose of Lipitor to 80mg daily. I developed huge problems with my gastrointestinal tract: I found it difficult to swallow, developed peptic ulcer disease and GERD, gastritis, and an hiatus hernia. My suspicions about Lipitor were not accepted by my doctors. Only when blood work came back with high CK levels did they tell me to stop taking Lipitor. Meanwhile, I was falling over with syncopes. On one occasion I fell down the porch steps and badly wrenched my leg. On others I fell down flights of stairs and hurt my back. I was given a tilt-table test which was positive for vaso-vagal syncope. All further symptoms of dizziness,

vertigo, nausea and fatigue were attributed to VV Syndrome. I had skull-splitting migraines, got hospitalized from life-threatening dehydration and had difficulty with transient loss of vision in one eye. I felt as if my feet were often standing in hot water, my fingers tingled and so did my toes. The slightest real exercise caused overwhelming muscle pain and overall fatigue. When I moved about the house it took me four days to get out of bed because I had no strength. My face sometimes felt numb in some areas, I experienced a loss of power in my hands. My heart developed leaks and regurgitation, sometimes it didn't beat as it should. By this time I had told the cardiologist who did my second catheterization that I thought statins were a huge contributory factor to my vascular problems. He told me to take Lipitor again. I did not do so because I thought it was a poison to my system. In the middle of 2003, having taken myself off statins, I started finding myself lost momentarily in familiar places. I forgot where I was going and why. I couldn't remember my telephone number or anybody else's. I received letters from people concerning letters and calls I made but did not remember making. My son brought in a trampoline that I had ordered by computer in the middle of one night. I don't have the strength to remove it from the box ! In December 2003 I fell down the stairs at 2 am one morning. I did not know why I was near the front door. Three hours later my son heard me fall down stairs again – this time I was fully dressed. It was 5 am but I thought it was afternoon. I told him I was going shopping. I was terrified that I was losing my mind. I went to see my doctor and he sent me for an MRI. It showed changes in the white matter of the left hemisphere of my brain. People noticed that I was slurring my words and couldn't make my mouth form the words properly. I saw a neurologist and he gave me Plavix. He said the arteries were going into spasm. He advised that I take a statin again because I have hypertension and many high risk factors. I was unsure. In March 2004 I had such bad chest pain that I went to the ER in the middle of the night. It was heartburn, two days later I had a 4 day episode of stroke like symptoms and Total Global Amnesia. I can't remember a thing but my family and friends were terrified that I couldn't stand or hold a cup to drink or feed myself; my manner changed and I became aggressive and insulting; I went in and out of total confusion. I demanded my car keys and fell down the stairs trying to get away. The doctor thought I'd experienced some sort of seizure or stroke. I totally lost 4 days. I saw more neurologists, they all said my symptoms were "bizarre." Nobody would consider a connection to statins, and to be truthful neither did I, because I had stopped taking Lipitor. Everybody was thrown by the fact that I gradually recovered though left with impairment of my short-term memory and language ability. I decided I'd had TIA's. I was advised to see a surgeon. Following my instincts, I found out about carotid surgery, and decided I didn't want anyone chopping on my neck, and went, instead, to a neuroscience center. Family and a friend came with me and they told the neurologist what they had seen when I had episodes. I brought up statins side effects; again I was assured these were not caused by Lipitor. I had MRI and MRA scans and EEG and transcranial Doppler testing. I was sent for a Neuropsychological test at the head injuries center.

Testing quantified the impairment. Frightened, I decided that I must have had a stroke. I taught myself to write with my left hand, with difficulty, because I can't hold things and make fine motor movements as well. My cholesterol level was above 400. My doctor told me I had to take a statin. I refused Lipitor but was persuaded to take Crestor at a 10mg daily level. I wasn't happy about that; but I was scared of having a major episode again and possibly never coming out of it. I was scared about going out on my own and of driving. I became more and more isolated from other people, as I felt "dumbed down." I used to teach history and had an excellent memory. I am 52 years old and, now, I couldn't remember what day it was or remember simple details from a story. I stopped watching television shows because I couldn't remember what had happened and was unable to follow the plots. I was very, very, frightened. Now, on Crestor, I couldn't sleep much and, when I did, I was woken by vivid dreams. My legs twitched and I felt short of breath. My kids admitted that I "was a shell of my former self." It was suggested that I apply for disability status. My gastroenterologist is currently doing testing on my GI tract. He said I probably have Multiple Sclerosis. I am horrified, because this was on top of uncontrolled FH and hypertension. I was even more anxious and depressed. I got on the websites about statins and I discovered Crestor was also regarded as "dangerous." What I then found out made me really, really, angry. Why were all the doctors discounting what all these people were saying about what had happened after they took statins? I called Pfizer, of which I am a shareholder, and their "product specialist" blew me off completely. They didn't even offer a biochemist or a physician, she was a nurse. I printed up a lot of stuff I found about statins and called the neurology center. My doctor said he had never seen anyone damaged by statin side effects. I said, " what about me?" When I tried to trace the course of my major problems in the last decade and a half I discovered that they fitted totally with statin side effects."

"I think that statins come with their own side effects but the drug can also trigger another illness in the patient. Getting worse may not be a function of the statin but a function of the other illness that was set off by the use of statins. We see that with Parkinson's and I am in contact with a few cerebellar ataxia where it is also true. These patients (and me) continue to get worse even after stopping the drug. It looks like statins act as a trigger for another illness. I just hope it is not fatal in the long run."

"Because Lescol wasn't affecting my cholesterol enough the doctor prescribed Lipitor and within months there was a drastic change. I developed a balance problem and walk with difficulty. I have slurred speech, a pain in my left knee when walking and a stiffness to my body when taking Lipitor. I have seen a neurologist who said I probably had cerebral insufficiency, an orthopedist who said I had arthritis, another orthopedist who said I didn't have arthritis and an internist who just doesn't know - all this after numerous x-rays and MRIs. For some reason I suspected the Lipitor and decided to stop it even though I knew the doctor objected. After two weeks the knee pain disappeared, my body stiffness was gone and I'm not as tired as I was. Walking is difficult still and my balance is not good. Also, my speech is still slurred and I don't feel as alert as I should be. Two months have gone by since I stopped the Lipitor and even though there has been some progress, I'm not sure there hasn't been irreparable damage."

"Today I finally received the following report from my doctor, which confirms what he told me: that my speech and swallowing difficulties were NOT caused by ALS, but probably were caused by Lipitor! I have included everything that he said except that I have not included his name. The neurologist, along with my speech therapist...and of course, me....were all ecstatic because of the encouraging EMG report.

My neurologist tells me that what has happened in my case is very rare indeed."

"I am interested in whether hand tremors have been listed as a side effect to Lipitor. My husband has been taking the drug for three plus years and just recently developed a rather coarse hand tremor, along with a stumbling walk. He has changed from rubber-soled shoes to leather ones due to frequent "tripping" episodes. His affect has changed from that of bright, attentive, humorous and insightful to one of flat and humorless. I have noted his driving skills have deteriorated, as well as other mechanical skills. He used to pride himself on being able to manipulate and solve mechanical problems, but now avoids anything mechanical. He also was a detail-oriented individual, who loved nothing more than following a set of complicated directions. Now he requests someone else read and follow the directions. He has begun to require more sleep than in the past and often takes a nap if time is available--something I have never seen him do in our 33 yrs. of marriage. I have thought of Parkinson's disease, but in discussing my concerns with my sister last evening, she related that her husband has begun exhibiting all these symptoms also, including the hand tremor! She too was concerned re: Parkinson's. Her husband was tested by a neurologist for both Parkinson's and Alzheimer's and both tests were negative. They live in one state; we live in another. Her husband and mine are of

similar age. They share one drug in common--
Lipitor! Could it be?"

"I was on Lipitor for three years; complained of
hand and stomach cramps to my doctor and stayed
on the drug; finally went to see a neurologist who
promptly diagnosed me with ALS and gave me three
to nine months to live. My sense is that Lipitor
affects the myelin sheath."

"I have often wondered if TGA is somehow
connected to Parkinson's. I am not sure how old
your article is on TGA. I have studied the web for
the past 5 years concerning TGA. My husband had
an attack in July of 2000. Your article on Lipitor
was the first time that I ever read of the relationship
between the drug and TGA. My husband used to be
on Lipitor before he was put on Pravachol and I do
believe that he was taking Lipitor at the time of his
attack. We will be going to his doctor on the 31st of
August and I am going to have them check his
records. He is now taking Zocor. My husband and I
were getting ready to go to the hospital to be present
at the birth of our son and daughter in laws first
baby. He went to take a shower and when he got out
he asked me where we were going. I thought he was
kidding. He didn't even remember that she was
pregnant. I of course thought he had a stroke and
called the paramedics. He was transported to the
same hospital where the baby was born. They told
us after many tests, that it was a classic case of
TGA. The doctor that he had at the time insisted that

he had a TIA but his neurologist confirmed in a subsequent visit that it was a TGA. After the TGA I noticed a difference in my husband. He was sent for a carotid artery study and many other tests. He has been diagnosed with Parkinson's disease for the past 2 years. I now wonder if this is true Parkinson's or if it could be caused by the meds. It is very frustrating to say the least. He has lost the use of his left hand and has had to take an early retirement."

"Yesterday I went up to the teaching hospital in my area and they said that I had MSA. A summary of MSA is: (Shy Drager syndrome) Multiple System Atrophy is a neurological disorder caused by degeneration of cells in certain areas of the brain. These control a number of different body systems; hence the name. They include functions of the autonomic nervous system (such as the control of blood pressure, sweating, bladder function) and the motor systems (such as muscle activation, movement and balance). MSA affects both men and women. Symptoms usually start between 40 and 60 years of age. The cause of MSA is not known, but is neither inherited nor contagious. I don't know anything for sure but I think that statins may have played a role in my developing this condition."

"I have read articles about side effects from Lipitor. I have taken other statins without major problems but after taking Lipitor for three years, my problems are almost identical to yours. My balance is bad,

writing is difficult, speech is slurred and motor skills diminished. I have seen neurologists, orthopedists, etc. and they came up with diagnosis of basilar insufficiency. They don't know for sure, however, just guessing. I can pinpoint when my walking, speech and imbalance started and they coincide to within a few months after starting Lipitor. I stopped Lipitor in Sept. 2004, and no longer have the muscle aches and stiffness but the other symptoms remain. I'm a 72-year old woman and too many problems are attributed to age. I was very active before but now activities outside the home are seriously curtailed and I now use a walker and no longer have pain."

"I am a polio survivor with diagnosed post polio syndrome, although I work full time in spite of it and don't appear disabled. I believe that because PPS is a neuromuscular disease that many drugs affect me adversely and I believe there is literature to prove this. I have a very high cholesterol level and at different physician's insistence I have tried a variety of cholesterol lowering medications. All have left me so fatigued I cannot function and I absolutely will not accept that. Four years ago a new family physician emphasized that I must take some sort of medication and so I agreed to take Lipitor. After several months I quit. I had severe fatigue and muscle aches. However because of PPS I can have these symptoms when I am overworked so I soldiered on and continued taking Lipitor as my doctor insisted. I finally gave up and discontinued

Lipitor. Within a week my fatigue greatly decreased and after 3-4 weeks my muscle aches disappeared. I did not return to my physician until several months later, at which time he threw up his hands in despair, so I agreed to try again. Of course I thought maybe my high stress job had caused the symptoms. But within 1 week of restarting Lipitor the muscle aches and fatigue returned. So, no more. I absolutely refuse to take any sort of cholesterol lowering medication. I will die from the side effects before anything else. Incidentally I am also an RN."

"I am 50 years old. In June 2002 I had a stent put in my heart (sorry I'm not sure where) and was immediately afterwards prescribed 80mg Lipitor daily. Everything was fine until December 2004 when I noticed partial vision loss in my right eye. The lower half of my vision in that eye looked as if I had looked at a bright light and looked away I can still partially see through it but with difficulty. Within a couple of weeks I became very anxious and depressed for no reason I could discern. I even had a full- fledged panic attack, which culminated with the feeling I was going to die on the spot. I went to my GP the next day and he was not able to find anything wrong with me. I also went to an optic neurologist who said he could find nothing wrong with the eye itself and an MRI and didn't find anything abnormal. Later he did a Visual Evoke Response test of which the findings were that there was some problem with the nerve, but he didn't

know what. The next test he wants to do is a spinal tap, which is scheduled for March 30th, but after finding this information this past Friday I'm thinking I might cancel that appointment. I have tried to contact my cardiologist but his nurse said I should just come in for an appointment, but that won't be until April 7th. I can't wait, I already am cutting my dose in half and will stay at that level for two weeks, my plan is to then cut it in half again for two more weeks, then go off altogether. Here is a complete list of all the symptoms I have noticed in the past 3 months: Partial loss of vision in right eye, Headaches, Depression, Anxiety, Fatigue, Tingling sensation in left arm and leg, Feeling pressure on the right side of my head, Left eye twitch, Muscle aches, Muscle Weakness, Muscle Cramping and Slight chest pain. By the way my last cholesterol report as of Jan 2005 was LDL 64, HDL 41, Total 117, Tri G 127, when I asked the nurse about reducing my dosage after getting those results she said that the only reason my readings were so good was the Lipitor and I should continue with my current 80mg dose. She also said the Doctor said I was still in, group B - whatever that means. I feel like I have been trapped in a prison, complete with a torture chamber. Until I found the many statin drug articles and stories on line this past Friday things looked pretty bleak, now I'm starting to see a light at the end of the tunnel - but it can't come soon enough! My Cardiologist so far has conveyed the notion that if I'm not on Lipitor I'm doomed. The way I feel right now I'd rather live shorter feeling good than a long time being miserable. I intend to continue take care of myself taking many natural supplements and continuing my exercising 5 to 6 times a week as I do now. I also am discovering how bad trans-fat is and will endeavor to avoid it as much as possible in the future. I have a feeling things aren't as bleak as my Cardiologist would suggest."

"My mom has been on cholesterol medication for almost 15 years. She is only 48 years old. The medicine she has been on ranged from all different types of statin drugs. The last being Zocor and then a switch to Vytorin. She has always suffered from stomach problems and then the last couple years she has noticed muscle weakening in her hands and cramping. After vigorously exercising regularly, the problems seemed to get worse. There is not much muscle left in her hands and she finds that her arms are very weak. Her muscles are easily tired and after a recent EMG she has noticed twitching throughout her body. She also seems to have slurring in her speech and difficulty writing. Basically the doctors are leaning towards ALS. I just have a hard time believing that this is the answer. Could it be possible that these really are side effects from the Statin Drugs?? Supposedly her EMG results were not great and the last doctor she saw seemed to think it was ALS. She has been off the statin drugs for 2 months now. Her symptoms are not any worse...they have pretty much stayed the same. I am so worried about her, but refuse to

believe that she has a life threatening disease. I'm just trying to get my mom back."

"I have also had a preliminary diagnosis of ALS. I am a 57-year old male and have been on Simvastatin (Zocor) for 12+ years at 60mg a day. My health care provider is the Veterans Administration. I am a medically retired pilot. Last Thanksgiving I thought at first I had had a stroke but over time I realized that this was no stroke as muscle weakness and movement were getting worse. A CT scan ruled out stroke so they sent me to a neurologist and he has made the preliminary diagnosis. I have an MRI, EMG and Nerve velocity test coming up. I have stopped taking Zocor (gradually) and it seems that symptoms have leveled off. Maybe wishful thinking but they are definitely not progressing at the rate they were. I am not getting any better at this time but not getting worse as far as I can see. The V.A. treats vets very aggressively and also had me on Metformin for borderline diabetes. My blood sugar was within national guidelines but not the V.A.'s. Without Zocor it seems my blood sugar is within their guidelines now without meds. Go figure."

"I have been on various statin drugs for 13 years. I have been on Zocor the most. About 2 years ago, the Dr. put me on Zocor and Zetia 20/10 mg. After a while, I started getting muscle cramps in my hands, legs, neck, and abdomen. I complained to the Dr. about it but he said to try and tolerate it because my

numbers were so good. About a year ago, he switched me to Vytorin. After about a month or two, I noticed that my hands were getting weak - I had difficulty with buttons and zippers and tying. Upon starting the Vytorin, I also started a vigorous exercise routine of running 4 miles 3 to 4 times a week and doing a boot camp routine. I then I noticed I had trouble doing lateral lifts with my right arm. I thought I had a weight lifting injury and then I thought I had carpal tunnel. Went to see my Dr. who noticed I had muscle atrophy between my thumb and index finger on my right hand. Thank God I'm left-handed. He sent me to a neurologist who did all the tests, MRI, EMG, nerve, etc. After the EMG, I started twitching all over. I couldn't even sleep. My mom suggested maybe I was having side effects from Vytorin, so I called my Dr. who said to stop taking it and see what happens. I stopped cold turkey. I would never recommend this. I had withdrawal symptoms of weakness, dizziness, vision problems, and twitching. I think you need to taper off gradually. The neuro said I was probably in the early stages of ALS. The EMG caused me to have a lot of twitching for 6-8 weeks. When I asked the neuro about it, he said that I was twitching before the test. I would have occasional twitches before but nothing like after that test. I ran 4 miles the morning of the test. I wonder if that could have contributed to the problem. Has anyone ever had twitching after the EMG? I have been off statins for about 4 months now. I haven't gotten any worse for which I am grateful. Whenever I overdo physically,

I pay for it. I no longer run---I do moderate walking and have given up weight lifting as it seems to cause weakness and twitching. I have been taking CoQ10 (1500 mg.) and other supplements. I have good days and bad days and try to keep a positive attitude. It's hard sometimes. On my last visit to the neuro, he was surprised at how strong I still am. He still thinks I am in the early stages of ALS but then added that he wouldn't "bet the farm on it". This comment gave me hope. He encouraged me to continue with my vitamins and supplements. I am also thankful to have discovered that ALS symptoms and statin toxicity are related. I have another EMG and neuro visit at U of MI Hospital scheduled in May."

REFERENCES

CHAPTER 1 – How the Statin Drugs Work?
1. Brousseau ME, Schaefer, EJ, *"Structure and mechanism of action of HMG-CoA reductase inhibitors "in HMG-CoA Reductase Inhibitors*, Schmitz, G., Torzewski, M, Eds. Basel, Schweiz, Birkhauser, 2002.
2. Shovman O and others. Anti-inflammatory and immunomodulatory properties of statins. *Immunol Res* 25(3): 272-85, 2002
3. Masato E and others. Statin prevents tissue factor expression in human endothelial cells. *Circulation* 105:1756, 2002
4. Chen F and others. New insights into the role of nuclear factor kB in cell growth metabolism. *American Journal of {Pathology* 159:387-397,2001
5. Hilgendorff A and others. Statins differ in their ability to block NF-kB activation in human blood monocytes. International *Journal of clinical pharmacology and therapeutics* 41(9): 397-401, 2003
6. Karin M, Delhase M. The 1 kappa B kinase and NF-kappa B: key elements of proinflammatory signaling. *Semin Immunol* 12(1): 85-98, 2000
7. Tato CM and Hunter CM. Host-pathogen interactions: subversion and utilization of the NF-kB pathway during infection. *Infection and Immunity* 70(7): 3311-3317, 2002
8. Raggatt LJ, Partridge NC. HMG-CoA reductase inhibitors as immunomodulators: potential use in transplant rejection. *Drugs* 62(15): 2185-91, 2002.
9. Kwak B and others. Statins as a newly recognized type of immunomodulator. *Nature Medicine* 6:1399-1402, 2000
10. Leung BP and others. A novel anti-inflammatory role for simvastatin in inflammatory arthritis. *J Immunol* 170(3): 1524-30, 2003
11. Palinski W Immunomodulation: A new role for statins? *Nature Medicine* 6:1311-1312, 2000
12. Ely JTA, Krone CA. A brief update on ubiquinone (Coenzyme Q10). *J Orthomol Med* 15(2): 63-8, 2000
13. Ely JTA, Krone CA. Urgent update on ubiquinone (Coenzyme Q10). (www.faculty.washington.edu/ely/turnover.html), 2000

14.   Langsjoen P, Langsjoen E. Statin associated congestive heart failure. *Proceedings of Weston-Price Foundation Meeting,* Spring, 2003.

15.   Langsjoen P, Langsjoen A. Coenzyme Q10 In cardiovascular disease with emphasis on heart failure and myocardial ischemia. *Asia Pacific Heart Journal* 7(3): 160-168, 1998.

16.   Gaist D and others. Statins and the risk of polyneuropathy: A case control study. *Neurology* 58: 1333-1337, 2002.

17.   Sparks S. Written personal communication. 8 August, 2003.

18.   Golomb B and others. Amnesia in association with statin drug use. *UCSD statin research study* (under review) 2002.

19.   Schwartz G and others. Effects of Atorvastatin on early recurrent ischemic events in acute coronary syndromes. *Journal of the American Medical Association* 285 (13): 1711-1717. 2002

20.   Sever PS and others. Prevention of Coronary and Stoke Events With Atorvastatin In Hypertensive Patients Who Have Average Or Lower-Than Average Cholesterol Concentrations in the Anglo-Scandinavian Cardiac Outcomes Trial. *Lancet* 361: 1149-1158, 2003

21.   The Allhat Officers and Coordinators For the Allhat Collaborative Research Group. Major Outcomes In Moderately Hypercholesterolemic, Hypertensive Patients Randomized to Pravastatin vs. Usual Care: The Antihypertensive and Lipid Lowering Treatment To Prevent Heart Attack Trial. *Journal of the American Medical Association* 288: 2998-3007, 2002.

22.   Collins R and others Heart Protection Study of Cholesterol Lowering With Simvastatin in 5963 People With Diabetes *Lancet* 361: 2005-2016, 2003

23.   Ravnskov U. *The Cholesterol Myths*, New Trends Publishing, 2000.

24.   Rosch Postdating drug side effects. *Proceeding of the Weston Price Foundation Meeting,* Spring 2003

25.   Matsuzaki M and others. Large scale cohort study of the relationship between serum cholesterol concentration and coronary events with low-dose simvastatin therapy in

Japanese patients with hypercholesterolemia. *Circ J* 66:1087-1095, 2002

26. Pfrieger F. Brain researcher discovers bright side of ill-famed molecule. *Science*, 9 November, 2001.

27. Muldoon MF and others. Effects of Lovastatin on cognitive function and psychological wellbeing. *Am J Med* 2000 May: 108(7) 538-460

28. Poole R, FAA headquarters, personal communication.

CHAPTER 2- Statins and Brain Cholesterol

1. Pfrieger F. Brainresearcher discovers bright side of ill-famed molecule. *Science*, 9 November, 2001.

2. Pfrieger, F. Ibid.

3. Muldoon MF and others. Effects of Lovastatin on cognitive function and psychological well-being. *Am J Med* 2000 May: 108(7) 538-460.........

4. Hodges JR, Warlow CP. The etiology of transient global amnesia: A case-control study of 114 cases with prospective follow-up. *Brain* 113: 639-657, 1990.

5. Wagstaff L and others. Statin associated memory loss: analysis of 60 case reports and review of the literature. *Pharmacotherapy* 23(7): 871-880, 2003.

CHAPTER 3 – Statins and CoQ10

1. Ely JTA, Krone CA. A brief update on ubiquinone (Coenzyme Q10). *J Orthomol Med* 15(2): 63-8, 2000

2. Ely JTA, Krone CA. Urgent update on ubiquinone (Coenzyme Q10). (www.faculty.washington.edu/ely/turnover.html), 2000.

3. Langsjoen P, Langsjoen E. Statin associated congestive heart failure. *Proceedings of Weston-Price Foundation Meeting, Spring, 2003.*

4. Langsjoen P, Langsjoen A. Coenzyme Q10 In cardiovascular disease with emphasis on heart failure and myocardial ischemia. *Asia Pacific Heart Journal 7(3): 160-168, 1998.*

5. Gaist D and others. Statins and the risk of polyneuropathy: A case control study. *Neurology 58: 1333-1337, 2002.*

6.   Phillip PS and others. Statin-associated myopathy with normal creatine kinase levels. *Ann Int Med* 137(7): 581-85, 2002
7.   Ely JTA, Krone CA. A brief update on ubiquinone (Coenzyme Q10). *J Orthomol Med* 15(2): 63-8, 2000.
8.   Wallace DC. Mitochondrial DNA in aging and disease. *Sci Amer 40-7.*
9.   Ibid.
10.   Wolfe S. Public citizen petitions FDA to warn doctors, patients about cholesterol drugs, 20 August, 2001
11.   Whitaker J. Citizens' petition filed with FDA to include coenzyme Q10 use recommendation in all statin drug labeling. *Life Extension Magazine, May 23, 2002*

CHAPTER 4 – Statins and Dolichols
1.   Griffiths G, Simons K. The Trans-Golgi Network: Sorting at the Exit Side of the Golgi Complex, *Science 243: 438-442, 1986.*
2.   Pert C. *Molecules of Emotion*, Scribner, New York, 1997
3.   Lambrecht BN. Immunologists getting nervous: neuropeptides, dendritic cells and T cell activation. *Respiratory Research 2: 133-38, 2001*
4.   Norris JF and others. *Neurosecretion: Retrospectives and Perspectives.* HW Korf and KH Usadel, Eds. Springer, Berlin, 71-85,1997
5.   Hokfelt T and others. General Overview of neuropeptides. The fourth generation of progress. (www.acnp.org/g4GN401000047/CH.html), 2000

6.   Golomb B and others. Severe irritability associated with statin cholesterol lowering drugs. *QJ Med.* 97:229-235. 2004.

CHAPTER 5 – Statins and nuclear factor kappa-B

1.   Shovman O and others. Anti-inflammatory and immunomodulatory properties of statins. (www.rheuma21st.com/archives/cutting_report_shoenfeld _antiinfl_statins.html) 10 December 2001
2.   Hilgendorff A and others. Statins differ in their ability to block NF-kB activation in human blood monocytes. *Internat J Clin Pharm and Therapeut* 41(9): 397-401,

2003

3. Karin M, Delhase M. The 1 kappa B kinase and NF-kappa B: key elements of proinflammatory signaling. *Semin Immunol* 12(1): 85-98, 2000

4. Masato E and others. Statins prevent tissue factor expression in human endothelial cells. *Circ* 103: 1736, 2002

5. Chen F and others. New insights into the role of nuclear factor kB in cell growth metabolism. *American Journal of {Pathology* 159:387-397,2001

6. Karin M, Delhase M. The 1 kappa B kinase and NF-kappa B: key elements of proinflammatory signaling. *Semin Immunol* 12(1): 85-98, 2000

7. Tato CM and Hunter CM. Host-pathogen interactions: subversion and utilization of the NF-kB pathway during infection. *Infection and Immunity* 70(7): 3311-3317, 2002

8. Raggatt LJ, Partridge NC. HMG-CoA reductase inhibitors as immunomodulators: potential use in transplant rejection. *Drugs* 62(15): 2185-91, 2002.

9. Kwak B and others. Statins as a newly recognized type of immunomodulator. *Nature Medicine* 6:1399-1402, 2000

10. Leung BP and others. A novel anti-inflammatory role for simvatatin in inflammatory arthritis. *J Immunol* 170(3): 1524-30, 2003

11. Palinski W. Immunomodulation: A new role for s statins? *Nature Medicine* 6:1311-1312, 2000

12. Ravnskov U. *The Cholesterol Myths*, New Trends Publishing, 2000.

13. Rosch P. Statin drug side effects. *Proceeding of the Weston Price Foundation Meeting,* Spring 2003

14. Matsuzaki M and others. Large-scale cohort study of the relationship between serum cholesterol concentration and coronary events with low-dose simvastatin therapy in Japanese patients with hypercholesterolemia. *Circ J* 66:1087-1095, 2002

CHAPTER 6 – The Role of Cholesterol in the body.

1.   Guyton AC, Hall JE. *The Adrenocortical Hormones.* In Textbook of Medical Physiology, 9th Ed, 957-971, Saunders, Philadelphia, 1996.
2.   Russel DW. Green Light for Steroid Hormones. *Science* 272: 370-371, 1996.
3.   Pfrieger F. Brain researcher discovers bright side of ill-famed molecule. *Science,* 9 November, 2001.
4.   Pfrieger, F. Ibid.
5.   Muldoon MF and others. Cholesterol Reduction and Non-Illness Mortality. Meta-Analysis of Randomized Clinical Trials. *British Medical Journal* 322: 11-15, 2001.
6.   Golomb BA. Cholesterol and Violence: Is There a Connection? *Annals of Internal Medicine* 128: 478-487, 1998.
7.   Wolozin B and others. Decreased Prevalence of Alzheimer Disease Associated With 3-Hydroxy-3-Methyglutaryl Coenzyme A Reduction Inhibitors. *Archives of Neurology* 57: 1439-1443, 2000.
8.   Golomb B. Statins and Dementia. Letters to the Editor, *Archives of Neurology* 58(7), July 2001.
9.   Pfrieger F. Cholesterol homeostasis and function in neurons of the central nervous system. *Cell Mol Life Sci* 60:1158-1171, 2003
10.   Lorin H. *Alzheimer's Solved.* Book Surge LLC, 2005
11.   Kaplan M. Low Cholesterol Causes Aggressive
12.   Behavior and Depression. *Psychosomatic Medicine* 56: 479-484, 1994.
13.   Bender KJ. Psychiatric Times 15(5), 1998.
14.   Duits N, Bos F. Depressive Symptoms and Cholesterol Lowering Drugs. *Lancet* 341, Letter, 1999
15.   Lechleitner M. Depressive Symptoms in Hypercholesterolaemic Patients Treated With Pravastatin, *Lancet* 340, Letter, 1999.
16.   Buydens-Branchey L, Branchey M. Association between low plasma levels of cholesterol and relapse in cocaine addicts. *Psychosomatic Medicine* 65: 86-91, 2003.
17.   Horwich TB and others. Low Serum total cholesterol is associated with marked increase in mortality in advanced heart failure. *Journal of Cardiac Failure* 8(4), 2002.
18.   McCully KS. *The Homocysteine Revolution.* Keats, 1997.

CHAPTER 7 – Role of inflammation in atherosclerosis

1. McCully KS. *The Homocysteine Revolution*. Keats, 1997
2. Pauling L. Unified concept of Cardiovascular disease. http://www.ourhealthcoop.com/pauling.htm
3. McCully K. Homocysteine theory of arteriosclerosis: Development and current status. In Gotto AM, Paolett R, editors, *Atherosclerosis Reviews* 11: 157-246, Raven Press, New York, 1983.
4. McCully K. Atherosclerosis, serum cholesterol and the homocysteine theory: A study of 194 consecutive autopsies. *American Journal of the Medical Sciences* 299: 217-221, 1990.
5. Wilcken DE, Wilcken B. The pathogenesis of coronary heart disease. A possible role for methionine metabolism. *Journal of Clinical Investigation* 57: 1079-1082, 1976.
6. Boushey CJ and others. A quantitative assessment of plasma homocysteine as a risk factor for vascular disease. *Journal of the American Medical Association* 274: 1049-1057, 1995.
7. Kauffman J. Should you take aspirin to prevent heart attack? *Journal of Scientific Exploration* 14 (4): 623-641, 2000.
8. Ravnskov U. *The Cholesterol Myths*, New Trends Publishing, 2000.

CHAPTER 8 – Our misguided war on cholesterol

1. Atkins, R. Dr. Atkins' *New Diet Revolution*. 3rd Ed. Evans, New York, 2002.
2. Taubes G. What If It's All Been A Big, Fat Lie? *New York Times Magazine*, July 7, 2002.
3. Eades MR, Eades MD. *Protein Power*. Bantam Books, 1996.
4. Sears B. *The Zone*. Harper Collins, 1997.
5. Steward H and others. *Sugar Busters*. Ballentine Books, 1998.
6. McCully KS, McCully M. *The Heart Revolution*. Harper Collins, 2000.
7. Willett W. Turning The Food Pyramid Up Side Down. *American Journal of Clinical Nutrition* 76: 1261-1271, 2002.

8. Enig MG, Fallon S. The Mediterranean Diet--Pasta or Pastrami? *The Weston A. Price Foundation Magazine,* Spring, 2000.
9. Ibid.
10. Keys A. Coronary heart disease in seven countries, *Circulation* 41(supplement 1), 1970.
11. Ibid.
12. Mann George. The great cholesterol scam. *21st century Science and Technology* 2(3), May-June 1989.

CHAPTER 9 – A failed national diet. What diet, then?

1. McCully KS, McCully M. *The Heart Revolution.* Harper Collins, 2000.
2. Banting, *Letter of Corpulence.* http://www.lowcarb.ca/corpulence/
3. Atkins RC. *Dr. Atkins' New Diet Revolution.* 3rd Ed. Evans, New York, 2002.
4. Kauffman J. Low carbohydrate diets. *Journal of Scientific Exploration, 2004.* (under review)
5. Braly J, Hoggan R. *Dangerous Grains: Why Gluten Cereal May Be Hazardous To Your Health.* Avery/Penguin Putnam, New York, 2002.
6. Ottoboni A, Ottoboni F. *The Modern Nutritional Diseases: Heart Disease, Stroke, Type-2 Diabetes, Obesity, Cancer, and How To Prevent Them.* Vincenti Books, Sparks, NV, 2002.
7. McCully KS, McCully M. *The Heart Revolution.* Harper Collins, 2000.
8. Bernstein, R. *Dr. Bernstein's Diabetes Solution.* Little, Brown, Boston, 1997.
9. Smith MD. *Going Against the Grain: How Reducing and Avoiding Grains Can Revitalize Your Health.* Contemporary Books, Chicago, 2002.
10. Allan C, Lutz W. *Life Without Bread: How a Low-Carbohydrate Diet Can Save Your Life.* Keats, Los Angeles, 2000.
11. Groves B. *Eat Fat Get Thin.* Vermilion, London, 1999.
12. Eades MR, Eades MD. *The Protein Power Lifeplan.* Warner Books, New York, 2000.
13. Atkins RC. Dr. Atkins' *New Diet Revolution.* 3rd Ed. Evans, New York, 2002.

14. Kwasniewski MD, Chylinski M. *Homo Optimus.* Wydawnictwo WGP, Warsaw, 2000
15. Enig M, Fallon S. The Oiling of America. *Nexus Magazine*, Feb-Mar, 1999.
16. McCully KS, McCully M. *The Heart Revolution.* Harper Collins, 2000.
17. Fallon S, Enig M. What causes heart disease? *Lancet* 1: 1062-1065, 1983
18. Kauffman J. Should you take aspirin to prevent heart attack? *Journal of Scientific Exploration* 14 (4): 623-641, 2000.

Chapter 10 - Statin Alternatives

Co-enzyme Q10 supplementation

1. Langsjoen P, Langsjoen E. Statin associated congestive heart failure. *Proceedings of Weston-Price Foundation Meeting*, Spring, 2003.
2. Langsjoen P, Langsjoen A. Coenzyme Q10 In cardiovascular disease with emphasis on heart failure and myocardial ischemia. *Asia Pacific Heart Journal* 7(3): 160-168, 1998.
3. Bargossi AM and others. Exogenous CoQ10 supplementation prevents ubiquinone reduction induced by HMG- CoA reductase inhibitors. *Mol Aspects Med.* 15(Suppl): S187-93, 1994
4. De Pinieux and others. Lipid-lowering drugs and mitochondrial function: effects of HMG-CoA reductase inhibitors on serum ubiquinone and blood lactate/pyruvate ratio. *Br J Clin Pharmacol.* 42(3): 333-37, 1996
5. Ely JTA, Krone CA. A brief update on ubiquinone (Coenzyme Q10). *J Orthomol Med* 15(2): 63-8, 2000
6. Ely JTA, Krone CA. Urgent update on ubiquinone (Coenzyme Q10), 2000 (www.faculty.washington.edu/ely/turnover.html)
7. Wallace DC. Mitochondrial DNA in aging and disease, *Sci Amer;* 40-7, 1997
8. Pauling L. Unified theory of heart disease. 1991 http://www.ourhealthcoop.com/pauling.htm

Omega 3 supplementation
1. Lee KW, Lip GYH. The Role of Omega-3 in the Secondary Prevention of Cardiovascular Disease. *Quarterly Journal of Medicine* 96: 465-480, 2003.
2. Omega-3 information service http://www.omega-3info.com/home.htm
3. Covington M. Omega-3 fatty acids. *AFP* 70(1) July 2004

The role of the B vitamins
1. McCully KS. The Homocysteine Revolution. Keats,1997.
2. Ubbink JB, *American Journal of Clinical Nutrition*, Jan 1993;57: 47-53
3. Selhub J and others. *JAMA* 270:2693-2698, 1993
4. Naurath HJ and others. *Lancet* 346:85-91, 1995

Why a buffered baby aspirin?
1. Kauffman J. *Malignant Medical Myths.* Infinity Publishing, 2005

Low dose statins
1. Matsuzaki M and others. Large scale cohort study of the relationship between serum cholesterol concentration and coronary events with low-dose simvastatin therapy in Japanese patients with hypercholesterolemia. *Circ J* 66:1087-1095, 2002
2. Hilgendorff A and others. Statins differ in their ability to block NF-kB activation in human blood monocytes. *Internat J Clin Pharm and Therapeut* 41(9): 397-401, 2003
3. Law MR and others. Quantifying effect of statins on low density lipoprotein cholesterol, ischaemic heart disease, and stroke: systematic review and meta-analysis. *BMJ* 326:1423, 2006
4. Shovman O and others. Anti-inflammatory and Immunomodulatory properties of statins. *Immunol Res* 25(3): 272-85, 2002

Mother Nature's statin

1.   Heber D and others. Cholesterol lowering effects of a proprietary Chinese red yeast rice dietary supplement. *American Journal of Clinical Nutrition 69:* 231-236, 1999.

Chapter 11 Conclusion

1.   McCully KS. *The Homocysteine Revolution*. Keats, 1997

2.   Pfrieger F. Brain researcher discovers bright side of ill-famed molecule. *Science,* 9 November, 2001

3.   Golomb B and others. Amnesia in association with statin use. UCSD College of Medicine, *Statin Research Study*, 2002 (under review)

4.   Cohen JS. *Over Dose, The Case Against the Pharmaceutical Companies,* Tarcher/Putnam, 2001

5.   Allred J. Lowering Serum Cholesterol: Who Benefits? 1993, *Journal of Nutrition* 123: 1453-1459, 1993.

6.   McCully KS, McCully M. *The Heart Revolution.* Harper Collins, 2000

7.   Lee KW, Lip GYH. The Role of Omega-3 in the Secondary Prevention of Cardiovascular Disease. *Quarterly Journal of Medicine* 96: 465-480, 2003.

8.   Langsjoen PH, Langsjoen AM. Overview Of The Use of Coenzyme In Cardiovascular Disease. *Cardiovascular Disease Biofactors* 9, (Issue 2-4): 273-285, 1999

9.   Kauffman JK. Should you take aspirin to prevent heart attack? *Journal of Scientific Exploration* 14 (4): 623-541, 2000.

10.   Sijbrands EJG and others. Mortality over two centuries in large pedigree with familial hypercholesterolemia: family tree mortality study. *BMJ* 322:1019-1023, 2001

11.   Collins R. Statin drug study of patients at high risk for heart disease. Oxford University, *American Heart Association,* 2001

12.   Jackson PR and others. Statins for primary prevention: At what coronary risk is safety assured? *British Journal of Clinical Pharmacology* 52: 439-446, 2001

12.   Schwartz GG and others. Effects of Atorvastatin on Early Recurrent Ischemic Events in Acute Coronary Syndromes. *Journal of American Medical Association* 285: 1711-1718, 2001.
13.   Simons J. PFIZER, The $10 Billion Pill. *Fortune*, 6 January 2003.
16.   Cohen JS. Over Dose, *The Case Against the Pharmaceutical Companies*, Tarcher/Putnam, 2001

ADDENDUM:

Genetic susceptibility and abnormal pathways of statin drugs' effects.

1.   Katirji B and others. Metabolic myopathies. *E Medicine* 2006
      http://www.emedicine.com/NEURO/topic672.htm
2.   Wang PY and others. OSBP is a cholesterol regulated scaffolding protein in control of ERK 1/2Activation. *Science*, 307:1472-76, 2005
3.   Meske V and others. *European Journal of Neuroscience*. 17: 93, 2003
4.   Chapman JM and Carrie A. Mechanisms of Statin-Induced Myopathy: A Role for the Ubiquitin-Proteasome Pathway? *Arterioscler Thromb Vasc Biol* 25: 2441-2444, 2005

What is your cardiovascular risk?
1.   Pauling L. Unified concept of Cardiovascular disease.
      http://www.ourhealthcoop.com/pauling.htm
2.   DNAprint Genomics, http://www.dnaprint.com

Mechanisms of Action of Transient Global Amnesia
1.   Lewis SL. Aetiology of transient global amnesia. *Lancet* 352: 9125,1998.

2. Homma S. PFO in cryptogenic stroke study. *Circulation* 105(22): 2625, 2002.
3. Richter F. Migraine aura and spreading depression. *Annals of Neurology* 49: 7-13, 2001.
4. Pfrieger F. Brain researcher discovers bright side of ill-famed molecule. *Science*, 9 November, 2001.

Statins and sexuality
1. Rizvi K and others. Do lipid lowering drugs cause erectile dysfunction? A systematic review. *Family Practice* 19 (1): 95-8, 2004
2. Adverse Drug Reactions Advisory Committee. Simvastatin and adverse endocrine effects in men. *Aust. Adverse Drug Reactions Bull* 14: 10, 1995
3. Bagheri and others. HMG CoA Reductase and erectile dysfunction: analysis of spontaneous reporting in France and Spain. www.pharmacol-fr.org/bordeaux2005/html/000299.html
4. Bruckert E and others. Men treated with hypolipidaemic drugs complain more frequently of erectile dysfunction. *J Clin Pharm Ther* 21(2): 89-94, 1996
5. L de Graff and others. Is decreased libido associated with the use of HMG-CoA-reductase-inhibitors? *B Clin Pharmacol* 58(3): 326-8, 2004
6. Jackson G. Simvastatin and impotence. *BMJ* 315: 31, 1997

Statins' neuro-degenerative effects?
1. Meske V and others. *European Journal of Neuroscience.* 17: 93, 2003
2. Lambourne S and others. *Molecular and Cellular Biology*, 2005 http://mcb.asm.org/cgi/content/abstract/25/1/278
3. Ferrer I and others, *Current Alzheimer's Research*, 2005 http://mcb.asm.org/cgi/content/abstract/25/1/278